Introduction to

Careers in Health, Physical Education, and Sport

Second Edition

Patricia A. Floyd
Alabama State University

Beverly J. Allen
North Carolina Central University

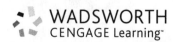

WADSWORTH
CENGAGE Learning™

Australia • Brazil • Japan • Korea • Mexico • Singapore • Spain • United Kingdom • United States

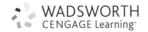

For product information and technology assistance, contact us at
**Cengage Learning Customer & Sales Support,
1-800-354-9706**

For permission to use material from this text or product, submit all requests online at **www.cengage.com/permissions**
Further permissions questions can be emailed to
permissionrequest@cengage.com

ISBN-13: 978-0-495-38839-5
ISBN-10: 0-495-38839-4

Wadsworth
10 Davis Drive
Belmont, CA 94002-3098
USA

Cengage Learning is a leading provider of customized learning solutions with office locations around the globe, including Singapore, the United Kingdom, Australia, Mexico, Brazil, and Japan. Locate your local office at:
international.cengage.com/region

Cengage Learning products are represented in Canada by Nelson Education, Ltd.

For your course and learning solutions, visit
academic.cengage.com

Purchase any of our products at your local college store or at our preferred online store
www.ichapters.com

Printed in the United States of America
1 2 3 4 5 6 7 11 10 09 08

CONTENTS

Part 4: On the Job

CHAPTER 1

CHOOSING YOUR CAREER

"The perfect job isn't a standard of living. It's a state of mind and state of being. In the perfect job, you're applying the talents you enjoy most to an interest you're passionate about, in an environment that fits who you are and what you value."

Leider and Shapiro

KEY CONCEPTS

1. The first step in career planning is self-assessment.
2. Proper preparation is necessary for a career in health, physical education and/or sport.
3. There are many career choices in health, physical education, and sport.
4. Setting goals/objectives is a critical element in choosing a career.
5. Making a career choice requires making major decisions.
6. Numerous resources offer services to assist in exploring and selecting a career.

INTRODUCTION

Choosing a career is a complex process. At this point it is very likely that you are anxious and even confused about choosing your career. Careers of today are very different than in the past and they will continue to change in the future. The demands of the twenty-first century have dictated changes in the structure of the workplace. There have been major changes in how we work, where we work, and how we prepare for work.

With the rapidly changing world of work, it can be difficult to make specific career plans for the near future, let alone for the rest of your life. However, it is important that you begin to clarify your career goals. One way to approach this important decision is to look at "what" you want to do and "where" you want to do it. The "what" addresses the skills you have or need to develop and the "where" relates to the environment in which you want to use those skills. You may be sure that you want a career in health, physical education, or sport, but you can't decide whether to pursue the traditional career and become a teacher or coach or to follow an alternative route and choose one of the non-traditional careers in the field. To clearly identify what you want to do and where you want to go, it is necessary for you to learn more about yourself and about the world of work. To begin the process, consider the following four critical questions:

- How do I plan for my career?
- Who am I?
- What are my career choices?
- What decisions do I need to make?

As you move forward in your career planning, avoid narrowing your choices of careers. In the past it was typical for students to complete a major related to a career, find a job in that field, and keep that job until they retired. Today, it is far more common for students to change their major and when they become employed, to make several career changes. Remember that there is no single right career out there waiting for you, but there are many career choices that you may find to be satisfying and fulfilling.

HOW DO I PLAN FOR MY CAREER?

Some of you may be sure of the career you will choose from the beginning, while even more of you will not be so sure and will change your mind numerous times before making a final decision. Thousands of people find satisfying careers each day while others have to change careers several times before they find a satisfying and fulfilling career. Your task is to figure out how you will choose a career(s) that matches your personality, values, skills, and interests. It will be necessary for you to take an in-depth and critical look at yourself, determine what your options are, and set your career goals. This is not the easiest of tasks and you may ask where you go for help. There are numerous resources available to you. Although you are ultimately responsible for your career planning, you will have the assistance of your academic advisor/counselor, career services personnel, and other resources such as professionals in the field to assist you along the way.

A visit with your academic advisor is a good place to begin. The academic advisor may be a full-time faculty member in your major area or a professional staff member in the advisement/counseling center. Whichever the case may be, your advisor will be able to give you advice on a variety of majors and careers, direct you in choosing courses that will meet both the requirements of your major and your personal interests, and assist you in developing your skills. Advisors in your major often have direct contact with agencies and organizations in the field and serve as contacts for internships, volunteer opportunities, employment referrals, and other prospective opportunities to gain experience and employment. Having a good relationship with your faulty advisor can open numerous doors for you. It is very likely that your advisor will suggest that you seek the services of the career services center to further research career fields that interest you and get additional assistance in planning your career.

The campus career services center located on your campus is an invaluable resource that offers a variety of career related services that are provided free of cost. Services include, but are not limited to, career counseling; administration and interpretation of assessments; workshops on decision-making, resume writing, interviewing; job fairs, and internship and career placements. A career counselor will assist you in assessing yourself, defining your interests, and setting your goals. Extended career services are available to help in structuring your career exploration and planning. These services include providing:

- Books, information and links to web sites that describe various career fields and occupations.
- A list of alumni who are willing to talk with you about their careers.
- Informational interviews to discuss potential careers.
- Opportunities for shadowing professionals in your career(s) of interest.
- Opportunities for internships and/or volunteer experiences.

Additional resources for assistance with planning your career are student organizations, upper class students, and mentors. Some student organizations focus on specific career interests. Upper class students can assist you in finding important resources. These students may have experience in the field and can share valuable information with you. Mentors can be upper class students or professionals already working in the career. There are countless ways that mentors can assist you in preparing for your career.

WHO AM I?

The career planning process begins with self-awareness. Self-awareness is a psychological-sounding term, but it means nothing more than knowing yourself. In other words ask yourself "Who am I?" Self-awareness can be accomplished through self-assessment, the process of gathering information about yourself. Self-assessment is a key factor leading to career success. Beginning with the self-assessment process can give you more insight and broaden your options. It will help you identify your strengths and your weaknesses. You can use the information to make informed decisions and have confidence that you are on the right career path. A complete assessment should include an analysis of your personality, values, skills, and interests. To prepare for this process, complete the University of Waterloo "Pride Experiences" exercise at http://www.cdm.uwaterloo.ca

Assessing Your Personality

Your personality is those distinctive individual traits and qualities that make you uniquely you. Your attitudes, needs, and motivations help make up your personality. Personality preferences affect what individuals are interested in and attract them to different lifestyles and careers. Understanding your personality is one of the most important factors in determining your happiness and success in a career and will help determine your career choices. The Myers-Briggs Type Indicator surveys basic personality traits and uses four scales to define eight personality preferences. The purpose of the inventory is to give you some indication of your personality preferences. There are no right or wrong answers and preferences have no relationship to your intelligence. Each individual possesses all eight preferences to some degree, but the identified area of preference is more pronounced. The personality preferences are:

- *Extroversion/Introversion*

    Persons with extroverted personality preferences are open and outgoing. They are attuned to the people, the culture, and their surroundings. Their strengths may include interacting well with people, openness, taking action and being easily understood. Their possible weaknesses may include the inability to work well without other people, impatience with routine, and impulsiveness. Those persons with introverted personality preferences are likely to be quiet and socially reserved. Their strengths are independence, reflectiveness, the ability to work well alone, and carefulness of actions. Weakness may include being misunderstood by others, secretiveness, avoidance of others, and missing opportunities to take action.

- *Sensing/Intuitive*

    Sensing persons prefer to deal with the facts. They think in detail and remember facts. Their strengths include being practical, systematic, and patient; paying attention to details; and having the ability to remember details and facts. Their weakness may be missing the "big picture," impatience with theory and the abstract, and mistrusting their intuition. Intuitive persons are open to possibilities. They take facts, look for relationships, and come out with broad concepts. Their strengths include the ability to envision possibilities, solve problems, work out new ideas, and be inspired. Possible weaknesses are impatience with routine, inattentiveness to details, jumping to conclusions, and losing sight of the present.

- *Thinking/Feeling*

    Thinking persons are logical and analytical. They make judgments based on evidence and avoid decisions based on empathy and values. Their strengths include their ability to be logical and analytical, organized, objective, critical but just, and making firm decisions. Weaknesses are the inability to be flexible, lack of compassion, disinterest in conciliation, misunderstanding of others' values, and the tendency to disregard others' values, feelings and needs. Feeling persons act on feelings, empathy, and values. They are interested in people. The ability to understand the needs and values of others, show their feelings, and consider others feelings are some of their strengths. In contrast, their weakness may be over acceptance of poor performance, lack of objectivity, less organization, and the lack of logic in decision-making.

- *Judging/Perceiving*

    Judging persons relate in a planned and orderly manner. They are decisive, sure and firm; making decisions and sticking to them. The ability to plan, make quick decisions, and remain on task is their strengths; while inflexibility, making decisions with insufficient data, stubbornness, and the tendency to be controlled by tasks or plans are weaknesses. Perceiving persons are flexible and spontaneous. They are open, nonjudgmental, and able to see and appreciate all sides of issues. Flexibility, compromise, and basing decisions on all the available information are strengths. Weaknesses are lack of control of circumstances, lack of planning, indecisiveness, easily distracted from tasks, and incomplete projects.

Assessing Your Values

The word values is defined by Gardner and Jewler as those important attitudes and beliefs that are accepted by choice, affirmed with pride, and expressed in action. The term may refer to specific beliefs that an individual holds on controversial and/or moral issues; to those things that are valued such as self-sufficiency, status, and accomplishment; or to the concepts of truth and justice. Values are those things that are most significant to you; those things around which you establish your priorities and for which you are willing to make a sacrifice. McKay identifies two types of values: intrinsic and extrinsic. Intrinsic values are related to the work itself and what it contributes to society. Extrinsic values include external features such as physical setting and earning potential. Your values influence your loyalties and your commitments. If you choose a career that is inconsistent with your values, it is very likely that you will dislike your work and will not be successful.

When you take a values inventory, your results may be compared with the Holland Self Directed Search system to find out where you fit in. Psychologist J. Holland developed a system of matching values with types of individuals and then matching the types with occupations. He ascribes people to the following six general categories based on differences in their skills, interests, values and personality characteristics, in other words, their preferred approaches to life. The categories are:

• *Realistic*

These people describe themselves as concrete, down to earth, and practical – as doers. They exhibit competitive/assertive behavior and show interest in activities that require motor coordination, skill, and physical strength. They prefer situations involving action solutions rather than tasks involving verbal or inter-personal skills, and they like to take a concrete approach to problem solving rather than rely on abstract theory. They tend to be interested in scientific or mechanical areas rather than cultural and aesthetic fields.

• *Investigative*

These people describe themselves as analytical, rational, and logical problem solvers. They value intellectual stimulation and intellectual achievement and prefer to think rather than to act, to organize and understand rather than to persuade. They usually have a strong interest in physical, biological, or social sciences. They are less apt to be people oriented.

• *Artistic*

These people describe themselves as creative, innovative, and independent. They value self-expression and relations with others through artistic expression and are also emotionally expressive. They dislike structure, preferring tasks involving personal or physical skills. They resemble investigative people but are more interested in the cultural aesthetic than the scientific.

• *Social*

These people describe themselves as kind, caring, helpful, and understanding of others. They value helping and making a contribution. They satisfy their needs in one-to-one or small group interaction using strong verbal skills to teach, counsel, or advise. They are drawn to close interpersonal relationships and are less apt to engage in intellectual or extensive physical activity.

• *Enterprising*

These people describe themselves as assertive, risk-taking, and persuasive. They value prestige, power, and status and are more inclined to other types to pursue it. They use verbal skills to supervise, lead, direct, and persuade rather than to support or guide. They are interested in people and in achieving organizational goals.

• *Conventional*

These people describe themselves as neat, orderly, detail oriented, and persistent. They value order, structure, prestige, and status and possess a high degree of self-control. They are not opposed to rules and regulations. They are skilled in organizing, planning, and scheduling and are interested in data and people.

Holland's system also organizes careers into the same categories based on the skills and personality characteristics most often associated with success in those careers and interests and values most often associated with satisfaction in the careers.

Adapted from John L. Holland, *Self-directed Search Manual* (Psychological Assessment Resources: 1985).

Assessing Your Skills

Skills assessment and development will be another important part of your self-assessment process. Skills are the things that you do well. They are under girded by aptitudes and can usually be improved with practice. Aptitudes are those strengths that are biologically inherent or the result of early training. Skills are the commodities that you offer and use in your career in exchange for your salary.

If you had to list your skills, how long would your list be? It probably would be short because you have not identified your skills and you are probably not accustomed to thinking and talking about them. Did you know that each person has more than 700 skills in their repertoire and that most people have a problem identifying them? Before you can move through a changing world of work, it is necessary for you to have a realistic look at your skills. In his book, *The Work of Nations*, Former Secretary of Labor, Robert Reich identified the following as basic work skills required by the new class of workers: abstraction, system thinking, experimentation, and collaboration.

Abstraction is the ability to discover patterns and meanings in order to make sense of the chaos of data encountered daily. System thinking is the ability to think in terms of the "big picture," to think of problems in the context of a complete system with interrelated elements. Experimentation is a skill that requires creativity and openness to chance. It addresses the ability to try something, evaluate the results, and make modifications until the desired results are achieved. Collaboration is the ability to work in a team effort. Collaboration is critical because of the interdisciplinary nature of work today and as the old saying goes, "Two heads are better than one." By interacting with others, it is much easier to discover new and innovative approaches to solving problems.

Thornburg researched five hundred job descriptions using a variety of web-based resources listed in the spring and summer of 2001. The research was restricted to full-time, non-apprentice positions from a wide range of industries. Six specific skills were mentioned as the most wanted workforce skills: technological fluency, communications skills, teamwork, leadership, problem solving, and creativity.

Over 80% of the jobs researched required technical fluency. Technical fluency is the ability to use computers and the Internet efficiently and comfortably. Employers expect employees to know which tools are best for which tasks, how to use them effectively, and how to deal with new versions of software o their own. Twenty five percent (25%) of the jobs researched required communications skills that go beyond the ability to write and speak well. Many of the descriptions mentioned proficiency with computer-supported presentation tools such as PowerPoint and incorporating other expressive modalities such as graphics and animation. teamwork (collaboration) was mentioned in 36% of the descriptions and implied in many more. Leadership was the fourth most wanted skill and, along with collaboration, was required at virtually every level of modern companies. Problem solving and creativity were implied in many of the descriptions. Successful applicants were described as those who had high tolerance for ambiguity, could problem solve, think "outside the box," demonstrate strong analytical skills, and learn new procedures, tools, and ideas quickly.

Similar to Thornburg, Lemke listed the following core skills necessary for the present-day worker:

1. Digital-Age Literacy
   • Basic scientific, mathematical, and technological literacies
   • Visual and informational literacies
   • Cultural literacy and global awareness

2. Inventive Thinking
   • Adaptability/ability to manage complexity
   • Curiosity, creativity, and risk taking
   • Higher-order thinking and sound reasoning

3. Effective Communication
   • Teaming, collaboration, and interpersonal skills
   • Personal and social responsibility
   • Interactive communication skills

4. High Productivity
   • Ability to prioritize, plan, and manage for results
   • Effective use of real-world tools
   • Ability to create relevant, high-quality products

In addition to the skills listed by Thornburg and Lemke, characteristics such as appreciation and understanding of cultural diversity, pride, and excellence were recurring themes in the web-based job descriptions.
Look at the following list of general skills that cut across all careers.

Leadership Skills

- Organizational skills and attention to detail
- Action-oriented and achiever of goals
- Customer/student focused
- Team-spirited; understanding of group dynamics
- Willingness to assist others
- Ability to take charge or relinquish control
- Mature, poised and personable
- Work cooperatively and collaboratively with different people
- Diversity awareness; all treated with respect and dignity

Interpersonal Skills

- Eager, professional and positive attitude
- Strong self-motivation and high self-esteem
- Confident and assertive, yet diplomatic an flexible
- Sincerity and integrity preserver
- Ambitious and risk taken
- Common sense
- Hard-working, disciplined and dependable

Communications Skills

- Good listener; compassionate and empathetic
- Good writing skills
- Excellent problem-solving and analytical skills
- Excellent oral communications skills
- Creative and innovative

Computer Skills

- Word processing
- Spreadsheet
- Database
- PowerPoint and presentation software

Adaptive Skills

- Quick learner
- Question seeker
- Analytical; independent thinker
- Willing to continue education and growth
- Committed to excellence
- Open-minded, willing to try new things
- Critical thinking/problem solving

Oriented to Growth

- Acceptance of an entry-level position; doesn't view required tasks as "menial"
- Academic excellence in field of study
- The organization's total picture viewed, not just one area of specialization
- Willing to accomplish more than required

Now, take a close look at the skills you possess. Determine your level of proficiency in those skills. Find ways to build on your strengths and to improve those skills in which you are less proficient. This will also help you identify the skills you are lacking and need to develop.

Assessing Your Interests

Interests are those things that you enjoy doing and they are key in making career choices. As your experiences and values change, your interests will continue to develop. Imagine having to go to work every day at a job in which you have no interest. What do you think your chances would be for achieving career success or satisfaction? Taking a more in depth look at your interests should provide insight about your interests and assist you in identifying careers that are compatible with your interests and that will keep you interested, enthusiastic and motivated. Interest inventories are often used in career planning as a means of gathering information about your interests.

There are a number of inventories/surveys available to help you learn more about yourself. These inventories should be helpful in assisting you with organizing and assessing the various aspects of yourself so that you can identify possible career choices. The inventories are generally available through your campus career center and many of them are available on the Internet. See Table 1.1 for a list of inventories.

As you take these inventories, keep in mind that they are not designed to dictate your career choices. If your results are different than you expected, you need only to develop interests and skills consistent with those required in the area of your choice. You are not bound to make decisions simply on the results of the assessments nor are you restricted from reversing those decisions.

Table 1.1 Inventories/Surveys

Personality Inventories/Surveys
Myers-Briggs Type Indicator Keirsey Temperament Sorter Personality Mosaic
Values Inventories/Surveys
Survey of Interpersonal Values Minnesota Importance Questionnaire Temperament and Values Inventory
Interest Inventories/Surveys
Holland Self-Directed Search Princeton Review Strong Interest Inventory

Practical and Related Experiences

Employers look for candidates with work experience and who have a fairly good understanding of what is involved in a job situation. The areas of health, physical education and sport offer an abundance of chances for you to gain valuable experience as you explore your possible career choices. Your college campus and the community offer a variety of programs and activities in which you can participate, allowing you to confirm or refute your interests, verify your values, and improve your skills. You can get experience through involvement in activities such as volunteer/service learning, internships/co-ops, clubs/organizations, additional coursework, study abroad, and employment.

Volunteer/service learning is an invaluable means of encountering real life situations, gaining practical experience, and helping others. These type activities are often required in courses and allow you to apply theory to actual practice. Such activities actively involve you in sharpening your teaming skills such as planning, problem solving, teamwork, and communication and relationship skills. The Secretary's Commission on Achieving Necessary Skills (SCANS) Report identified foundational skills and competency areas that are required in the workplace. Of those skills and competencies, volunteer/service learning contributes to the development of:

- basic skills - language arts and math
- thinking skills – making decisions, reasoning, creative thinking, problem solving
- personal qualities – integrity, honesty, responsibility, sociability
- resources – identifies, organizes, plans, and allocates resources
- interpersonal – understands complex relationships
- technology - works with a variety of technologies

Gardner identifies eight behaviors essential for leaders in *Self-Renewal: The Individual and the Innovative Society*. Volunteer/service learning requires the use of these behaviors and contribute to their development. The behaviors are:

- strengthening the vision, ability, and skills of followers
- unlocking and channeling energy which motivates
- achieving workable unity
- identifying, exploring, interpreting, and clarifying new directions, initiatives, and goals
- representing the group
- staying informed and sharing information and power
- removing barriers
- locating and mobilizing resources

Volunteer/service learning provides opportunities to serve others and learn simultaneously and can be both professionally and personally rewarding. Examples of different volunteer/service learning roles include:

- tutoring
- mentoring
- assisting teachers
- working with the aging
- sponsoring food drives
- helping in hospitals
- assisting with health related community projects
- working with disabled students
- coaching sports
- teaching sports
- working with community organizations
- working with professional organizations
- working with business organizations

Internships/co-ops are meaningful experiences within the professional workplace that allow you to learn, understand, and practice the skills and competencies needed to succeed and network with employers and employees within the workplace. In addition, these activities allow you to determine whether the career meets your interests, expectations and goals.

Clubs and professional organizations are a source of information that also provide opportunities to use and develop you leadership and interpersonal skills. Participation in these clubs and organizations will give you insights into careers, help you network with other students with similar career interests, and keep you abreast of possible internship, volunteer, and other career related opportunities.

Additional coursework is a good way to increase your skills and knowledge base. Public speaking, writing, and other similar courses may be taken to enhance your basic skills. Technology and other specialized courses can be taken for exposure to a variety of skills and knowledge. Be sure to check for prerequisites before enrolling in specialized courses.

Study abroad can be an exciting way to gain experience and learn from a global perspective. Study abroad can assist you in learning about different cultures and adapting to different traditions. Globalization is expanding opportunities for careers around the world, as well as presenting the possibility of working with others from countries.

Employment is an excellent means of building your skills and experiencing work environments. On or off campus employment, full time or part-time, employment gives you a chance to practice good work habits and provide experience in communication, time management, interpersonal and other skills that employers are looking for in employees.

Goal Setting

You can take charge of your life! Taking charge of your life requires that you do something more for yourself than just have feelings, intentions and thoughts. It requires that you set goals and carry them out. Psychologists such as Abraham Maslow believe there is an innate drive in all of us that propels us to be our best. Failure to reach our potential can lead to frustration, unhappiness, and despair. Setting personal goals are a direct way to prepare for your career and make a positive difference in your life.

Goal setting is an "action." It is something you want to do to better yourself or your life situation. Goal setting means that you take action. The pursuit and achievement of long-range goals provides direction, purpose and satisfaction in life. Long-term goals are the destination or final place you want to end up and short-term goals are the small steps you take along the way to achieving your long-term goals. You need motivation and a plan. How can you hit a target you don't have? It is just as difficult to reach a destination you don't have, as it is to come back from a place you have never been. People who don't succeed in life don't plan to fail. They simply don't plan anything. True there is some danger in setting goals, but the risk is greater when you don't set goals. J.C. Penny once said: "Give me a stock clerk with a goal and I will give you a person who will make history. Give me a person without a goal and I will give you a stock clerk."

> "Obstacles are things a person sees when he/she takes his/her eyes off his/her goals."
>
> Anonymous

Set Performance Goals

When setting goals you should have as much control over the achievement of your personal goals as possible. Goals based on outcomes are extremely vulnerable to things beyond your control. When you base your goals on personal performance targets or skills to be acquired, you can keep control over the achievement of your goals and receive satisfaction from accomplishing them.

Set Specific Goals

You should set goals that are specific and measurable. Setting specific goals will help you identify exactly what you want to achieve. Your goals must also be measurable. Setting measurable goals will allow you to see what you have accomplished and what remains to be accomplished.

Set Realistic Goals

Your goals should be realistic but challenging. They should be slightly out of your immediate grasp, but not so far that there is no hope of achieving them. If you find that you are consistently failing to meet your measurable goals, analyze the goals and adjust them to meet your needs. By setting goals effectively you can achieve and maintain strong forward momentum.

"You are not finished when you fail. You are finished when you quit."
Anonymous

Set Self-Referenced Goals

Focus your goals on yourself and your personal achievement. You have no control over what others do, but you do have control over what you can do. In other words, your goals must fit you and meet your needs.

Go ahead and set your goals. Write them down and come up with a plan for achieving them. Your plan will involve identifying and implementing small concrete steps so that you make progress every day, no matter how small, toward your goals. Seeing the results will provide you with confidence that will enable you to achieve even higher and more difficult goals.

Figure 1.1   Career Goals

Goal # 1	
Goal #2	
Goal #3	

WHAT ARE MY CAREER CHOICES?

There are many types of careers in health, physical education and sport. If you do some research you will discover that careers in the areas of health, physical education and sport are increasing at a phenomenal rate.

Figure 1.2 Careers

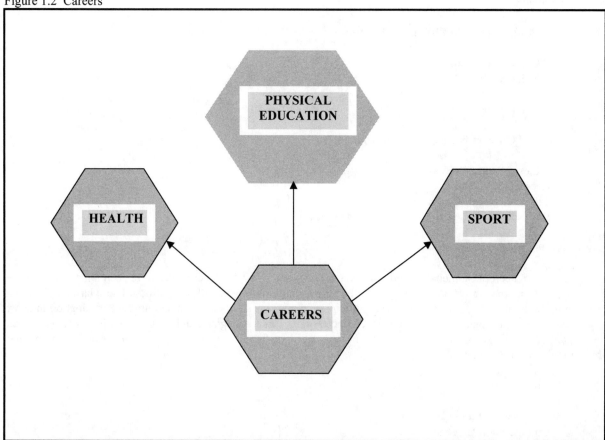

Career Opportunities in Health

Health occupations continue to grow and required skilled employers with all types of knowledge, skills, abilities, and interests. There are a wide variety of careers ranging from a health teacher, to biomedical equipment personnel, to administrator, and to basic health care and preventive medicine. Types of career opportunities that in health include:

- **Teaching Careers in Health**

  - 6-12 School Careers
  - Specialized Post Secondary Careers
  - Post-Secondary Careers

- **Related Careers in Health**

  - Public and Community Health Careers
  - Therapy-Related Careers
  - Professional Association/Organization Careers

Career Opportunities in Physical Education

Career opportunities in physical education have become progressively more diverse over the past four decades. A wide variety of careers ranging from physical education teacher, to recreation specialist, to researcher, to administrator and many more in between are available. Types of career opportunities that are available in physical education include:

- **Teaching Careers in Physical Education**

  - PK-12 School Careers
  - Specialized PK-12 School Careers
  - Post-Secondary School Careers
  - Specialized Post-Secondary Careers

- **Related Careers in Physical Education**

  - Fitness/Health Careers
  - Recreation Careers
  - Therapy-Related Careers
  - Professional Association/Organization Careers

Career Opportunities in Sport

Sport has experienced phenomenal growth on every level over the last forty years. We have seen a marked increase in participation in sport by children and youth, the aging, and individuals with disabilities. There has also been an increase in the number of aging citizens who participate in amateur sports through activities. Participation in sport has also experienced tremendous growth on the interscholastic, intercollegiate, and professional levels. This growth trend is reflected in the increase in the variety and availability of sport careers. Types of career opportunities that are available in sport include:

- **School Sport Careers**

  - High School Sport Careers
  - College Sport Careers

- **Professional Sport Careers**

  - Professional Teams
  - Associations & Organizations
  - Broadcasting & Media Sport Careers
  - Sports Events Careers
  - Sporting Goods Careers
  - Professional Services Sport Careers

Chapter 2 Introduction to Careers in Health, Chapter 3 Introduction to Careers in Physical Education, and Chapter 4 Introduction to Careers in Sport will familiarize you with a broad scope of diverse career opportunities in each respective area. A thumbnail profile including responsibilities, qualifications, and general salary range for selected careers in each area is presented. Examine the range of career options in each of these chapters; determine which career(s) are suited to your interests, aptitudes, and experiences; then explore.

WHAT DECISIONS DO I NEED TO MAKE?

Now that you have done the research, it is time to make some decisions. Making decisions is the process of making a choice to follow one course of action as opposed to another. Will you seek employment as a teacher? Will you choose a nontraditional career? Will you continue your education? What courses should you take? Will you start your own business? Career related decisions in terms of career choices and preparations have to be made. What do you want to do and what do you need to do in order to do what you want to do?

The decisions you make should be based on information that you have gathered and on the vision of how you see yourself in the future. Be mindful that your decisions always result in action. Making a choice to do nothing is also a decision that results in the selection of a course of action.

As you begin or continue the process of exploring and making the important decisions relative to selecting the right career for you, keep in mind the following dos and don'ts.

Do:

- Explore numerous opportunities related to your field of study by volunteering, joining student organizations, and taking internships and co-ops.
- Explore with your career counselor, faculty advisor, mentor, employers and other individuals the number of career possibilities.
- Meet regularly with your academic major advisor.
- Seek what you enjoy doing and just do it!

Don't:

- Choose courses because your family or others suggest them. That will be a waste of your time, energy and money.
- Seek a career for monetary gains or prestige. Seek a career that you have a passion for, a career that will cause you to love going to work each day.
- Limit yourself to courses required in your major. Broaden your potential by taking additional courses, especially technology, to make yourself marketable in various careers.

Take Action!

- Make an appointment to see your academic advisor/counselor. Visit on a regular basis to discuss your major, your coursework, your career interests, plans, and decisions, and your career options.

- Visit your on-campus career services center to discover career options, refine your career plans, and take advantage of the many other services offered.

- Take a variety of self-assessment inventories to help evaluate your personality, interests, values, and skills.

- Attend resume writing, interviewing, and other job search skills workshops sponsored by your career services center.

- Take a variety of courses to get exposure to knowledge and skills in a variety of areas, to improve your communication skills including: oral, written, listening, and technology skills, and to increase your critical thinking and problem solving skills.

- Volunteer or get a job in order to get experience, explore careers, and help others.

- Become a member of clubs and organizations in and out of your school and work to develop your interpersonal and leadership skills.

- Network with friends, instructors, family, and acquaintances to gain information in your area of career interest.

- Use a variety of resources such as Internet, career services center, library, chambers of commerce, newspapers, and phone books to conduct research on careers options.

- Seek opportunities to observe employers on the job in your career area of interest. Also, request informational interviews to explore career opportunities with these employers.

- Prepare a draft of your resume and ask your career counselor and academic advisor/counselor to review it and make comments.

- Explore overseas study possibilities to gain a global perspective on career options.

- Attend career fairs to network with employers and set up interviewing opportunities for internships and other career-related opportunities.

- Explore graduate school as an option for further career preparation.

The process of making a career choice involves all of the action items listed above. You do not have to do all of these things at once and there is no specific order in which they must be done. These actions are designed to help you develop your knowledge and skills, make good decisions, and to be actively involved in opportunities on campus and in the community. Keep your career goals in mind, but remain open for opportunities that you don't expect.

Think about your present situation and what you have done so far to begin to plan your career. Place a check next to the statements that best describe actions you have already taken. If there are items with no response, make these actions a priority.

1. _____ I have made contact with my academic advisor.
2. _____ I have visited the career service office at my college/university.
3. _____ I have selected a major and know the various career opportunities.
4. _____ I have selected a major but am not sure if it is the right choice for me.
5. _____ I have selected a major that I enjoy.
6. _____ I have the necessary skills and abilities to lead to my career of choice.
7. _____ I know how to compose different types of resumes.
8. _____ I know how to write a cover letter to accompany my resume.
9. _____ I have discussed the advantages/disadvantages of my selected career with a professional in the career.
10. _____ I am willing to remain open to new career opportunities.
11. _____ I have visited an agency/organization and have observed professionals in my area of interest at work.

SUMMARY

Being successful and satisfied in your career is an accomplishment that each of us wishes to achieve. But to do so requires proper preparation and planning. There are many resources available to assist you with this task. Take full advantage of them. Learn more about yourself in terms of your personality, values, skills, and interests and use the information to make informed career choices. Set your career goals and go for it. Remember that you are seeking a career, not just a job. A job is what you do with your days; a career is what you do with your life.

REFLECTIONS

1. What are your career goals? List five goals that you set for yourself. Review the goals that you have listed and circle the five you want the most. Rank them by priority – 1 for most important, 5 for least important. Be prepared to discuss your choices in class.

2   After completing the inventory in Activity Laboratory 1.1, reflect on what you have learned about yourself Discuss how this inventory is similar or different from your perception of your personality.

3. After completing the inventory in Activity Laboratory 1.2, reflect on what you have learned about yourself Discuss how this inventory is similar or different from your perception of your interests.

WEB SITES

www.advancingwomen.com/awcareer.html
Advancing Women Career Center

http://careerplanning.about.com
Career Planning

www.careers.org
Career Resources Center

www.jobweb.com
Career Selection

www. self-directed-search.com/taketest.html
Holland Self-Directed Search

www.jobweb.com
National Association of Colleges and Employers

www.bls.gov/oco/
Occupational Outlook Handbook

www.peterson.com/
Peterson's Web site

www.review.com
Princeton Review

www.keirsey.com
Keirsey Temperament Sorter

www.testingroom.com
self-assessment

BIBLIOGRAPHY

Bardwell, C.B. (1998*).* How to evaluate a job offer. *The Black Collegian,* 28:2. 64-68.

Bolles, Richard Nelson; Christen, Carol; and Blomquist, Jean M. (2006). *What Color is Your Parachute ?:*
     For Teens, a Practical Manual for Job-hunters and Career Changers. Berkeley, CA: Ten Speed Press.

Brown, M. (1997*).* Globalize yourself. *Next Step*, 2:2, 50-52.

Floyd, P.A. and Allen, B.J. (2008). *Professional Development for Pre-Service Teachers, 2*[nd] *ed.* Boston , MA:
     Pearson Education.

Gardner, W. (1995). *Self Renewal: The Individual and Innovative Society*. New York: W. W. Norton.

Gardner, J.N. and Jewler, A.J. (2006). *Your College Experience Strategies for Success*, Media edition, 6th ed.
     Belmont, CA: Wadsworth/Thomson Learning.

Harr, J.S. and Hess, K.M. (2006). *Careers in Criminal Justice and Related Fields: From Internships to*
     Professionalism, 5th ed. Belmont, CA: Wadsworth/Thomson Learning.

Job Choices: A Guide To The Job Search For New College Graduates, 46[th]ed. (2003). National Association of
     Colleges and Employers, Bethlehem, PA.

Leider, R.J. and Shapiro, D.A. (1996). *Repacking Your Bags: Lighten Your Load For The Rest Of Your Life*. San
     Francisco: Berrett-Koehler Publishers.

Lemke, C. (2001). 21st Century Skills. www.ncrel.org/engauge/skills/skills.htm.

Reich, R. (1992). *The Work of Nations: Preparing Ourselves for 21*[st]*-Century Capitalism*. New Your: Vintage
     Books.

Ryan, R. (2008). *The Dream Maker with "What to do with the Rest of Your Life."* www.robinryan.com

Swick, J., Winecoff, H., Rowls, M., Kemper, R., Freeman, N., Mason, J., Janes, D., and Creech, N. (2001).
     Developimg Leadership in Faculty and Students: The Power of Service Learning in Teacher Education. South
     Carolina Department of Education.

Thornburg, D. (2002). *The New Basics: Education and the Future of Work in the Telematic Age.* Alexandria, Va.:
     Association for Supervision and Curriculum Development.

LABORATORY ACTIVITY 1.1

NAME _____ DATE _____

COURSE _____ SECTION _____

Complete a personality inventory such as the Myers-Briggs Type Indicator or the Keirsey Temperament Sorter www.keirsey.com at your career services center or on the Internet. Reflect on what you have learned from the instrument. Discuss how this inventory is similar or different from your perception of your personality.

LABORATO8885RY ACTIVITY 1.2

NAME _____ DATE _____

COURSE _____ SECTION _____

Complete an interest inventory such as the Princeton Review Career Quiz (www.review.com) or the Holland Self-Directed Search (www. self-directed-search.com/taketest.html). List your top five occupational interests based on the inventory. Discuss how this inventory is similar or different from your perception of your interests. Use Laboratory 1.2 for your response.

LABORATORY ACTIVITY 1.3

NAME _____ DATE _____

COURSE _____ SECTION _____

Complete a values inventory such as the Minnesota Importance Questionnaire (psych.umn.edu/psyy/lab/vpr/miqing.htm)at your career services center or on the Internet. Reflect on what you have learned from the instrument. Discuss how this inventory is similar or different from your perception of your values.

CHAPTER 2

INTRODUCTION TO CAREERS IN HEALTH

"No knowledge is more crucial than knowledge about health…Without it; no other life goal can be successfully achieved."

Carnegie Foundation Report on Secondary Education in America

KEY CONCEPTS

1. Careers in health can be divided into four subcategories: health promotion, medical care and treatment, medical technology, and health information management and support services.
2. Health promotion encompasses the broad scope of the process of enabling people to increase control over and improve their health.
3. Health education is learning which enables individuals to make decisions and modify conditions to enhance health.
4. There are many diverse careers in the areas of medical care and treatment, medical technology, health information management and support services.

INTRODUCTION

Of all the industries experiencing economic growth in our nation today, none is growing more rapidly than the health care industry. There are many diverse health and health related professions. The U.S. Department of Labor/Bureau of Labor Statistics has categorized health careers into the following two major occupational groups.

- Health Care Practitioners and Technical Occupations
- Health Care Support Occupations

The major categories have been further divided by the authors into secondary categories for easy identification and reference. Many of the selected careers can be cross-referenced, as they may well fit into other categories, but have not been so treated in this text. Secondary categories of health careers include the following areas of classification.

- Health Promotion
- Medical Care and Treatment
- Medical Technology
- Health Management and Support Services

Figure 2.1 Health Careers

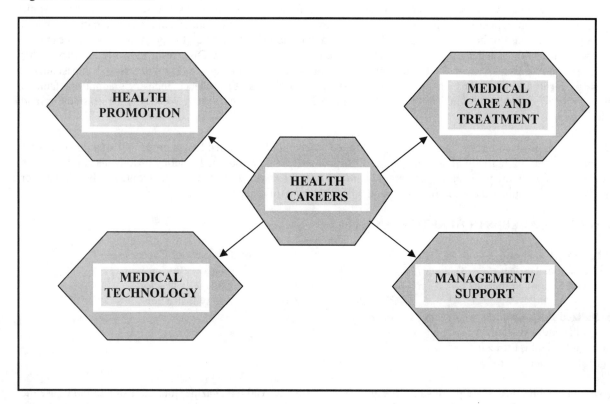

What is Health Promotion and Health Education?

Health promotion is the process of enabling people to increase control over and to improve their health. The term health promotion is defined by the Joint Committee on Health Education Terminology as "the aggregate of all purposeful activities designed to improve personal and public health through a combination of strategies, including the competent implementation of behavioral change strategies, health education, health protection measures, risk factor detection, health enhancement and health maintenance." Health promotion is broader in scope than health education and health education is an intricate part of health promotion.

Health education as stated by the Joint Committee on Health Education Terminology is a "continuum of learning which enables people, as individual members of social structures, to voluntarily make decisions, modify, and change social conditions in ways which are health enhancing." Green and Kreuter defined health education as "any combination of learning experiences designed to facilitate voluntary actions conducive to health."

Health education can be used to influence health and quality of life for people. From the teacher's perspective, health education is the process of developing and providing planned learning experiences to supply information, influence behavior, and change attitudes. In fact, candidates should develop a sense of individual responsibility for their health, leading to health enhancement or high-level wellness. Candidates should develop self-esteem, self-confidence, and a sense that he or she can achieve success not only in health-related matters, but life in general.

What is Community and Population Health?

In order to understand the careers in health education one must first understand community and population health. Community health refers to the health status of a community and to the organized responsibilities of school health, public health, transportation, safety, and other tax-supported functions, with private and voluntary actions, to promote and protect the health of local populations identified as communities. Population health refers to the health status and the conditions influencing the health of a category of people (women, adolescents, prisoners) whether the people define themselves as a community or not. A population could be a segment of the community or several communities of a region.

The purpose of Community health is to blend the influences of public health, school health, occupational health, social and recreational services, mass media, housing, transportation, mutual aid and self care in the service of whole populations. The growing recognition of categories of health of people who do not constitute communities, either in the geographical sense or in the organizational sense cause the addition of the title of population health. An example of population health includes the British government report on the Mad Cow Disease in its cattle industry. This report spooked consumers over food safety more than outbreaks of salmonella in hamburgers and unpasteurized juices in North America. The population health "story" of 1997 was the tobacco industry's admitting fault in tobacco-related deaths. Additional developments include Dolly, the cloned sheep, West Nile virus, smoking and pollution.

New directions for health came in 1990 with the Surgeon General of the United States proposing a national plan for promoting health among individuals and groups. *Healthy People 2000* outlined a series of long-short-range goals and objectives. Like the preceding document, *Healthy People 2010* will serve as the cornerstone and benchmark for what is to be accomplished concerning the nation's health during this decade.

TEACHING CAREERS IN HEALTH EDUCATION

6-12 School Careers
Middle School Teacher (6th – 8th grade)
Secondary School Teacher (9th – 12th grade)

Post-Secondary School Careers
Junior College Instructor
Community College Instructor
College/University Instructor

Specialized Post-Secondary Careers
Personal Health Professor
Community Health Professor
Occupational Health Professor

Careers in teaching health are promising. It is almost impossible to read a magazine, journal, listen to radio, use the Internet, or watch television without extensive information on some health-related issue, topic or activity. As health education teachers, the responsibility is to motivate candidates to improve their own health status through positive self-direction. Health education offers candidates and opportunity for personal growth and enhancement that is not duplicated anywhere else in the curriculum. Choosing a career in health education can provide you the opportunity to enhance the health promotion movement for all Americans.

Education and Practical Experience

To become a teacher in the traditional school health education setting requires a minimum of a bachelor's degree. Individuals must meet entry level requirements to enter the profession. Many states require teacher preparation candidates to pass a standardized examination and achieve on a 4-point scale a 2.5 or better cumulative grade point average to gain admission to and maintain retention in the program. There may also be other requirements such as receiving a passing score on reading and writing proficiency exams. A 2.5 or better grade point average must be maintained cumulatively, and in both the content area and the professional studies area to enter the professional internship. An exit examination may also be required for completion of the program. The exit examination may include teaching a demonstration lesson, a portfolio, a written examination, an interview or any variety of related activities. Upon completion of your curriculum and meeting requirement, you will enter the final phase of preparation for entry into the teaching profession: the professional internship. Examples of the types of courses required in general studies, the content area, and in professional studies are listed in Table. 2.1.

The health education curriculum in Table 2.1 is an example of typical health education teaching course requirements and professional content health education courses for a basic teacher certification program. Universities may require different courses and different numbers of hours for the completion of the program. Refer to your college/university catalog and check with you academic advisor for requirements specific to your program.

In addition to the satisfactory completion of coursework, employers seek candidates with work experience and who have a good understanding of what is involved in the job situation. The professional internship is required and is one means of attaining some formal experience. It is an opportunity for you to see how it feels to be a teacher in a real teaching environment. The internship may last anywhere from twelve weeks to one year. Outside of classroom experiences required in the curriculum, there are numerous opportunities for you to gain valuable applicable experiences. Volunteerism is an excellent way to gain valuable experience. There are opportunities to give of your time in community agencies such as American Heart Association, American Cancer Association, hospitals, school health programs local and, public health departments. There are also opportunities for part time and summer jobs that will give you invaluable experiences and great additions to your resume.

Table 2.1 Health Education Curriculum

General Studies	Content Area	Professional Studies

English Composition
Introduction to Literature
Humanities (e.g. Art Appreciation)
History
General Psychology
World Geography
General Biology
Physical Science
Mathematics
Speech
Personal Health
Orientation
	Introduction to Health Education
	Consumer Health
	First Aid and CPR
	Human Anatomy & Physiology
	School and Community Health
	Health and Nutrition
	Alcohol and Drug Education
	Human Sexuality
	Community and Chronic Diseases
		Foundations of Education
		Psychology of Learning
		Test, Measurement, and Evaluation
		   Health and Physical Education
		Instructional Technology for
		   Educators
		Classroom Management
		Methods of Teaching Elementary
		   School Health Education
		Methods of Teaching Middle/High
		   School Health Education
		Reading in the Content Area
		Diverse Students in Inclusive
		   Schools
		Professional Internship in 6-12 in
		   Health Education

Professional Competencies

The characteristics of an outstanding educator are similar whether it is a health education teacher and or a regular classroom teacher. A teacher must have the ability to relate positively to others, enjoy young people, have a commitment to the teaching process, continue in professional development activities, and to have the ability to motivate others.

Personal characteristics include: communication skills, honesty/integrity, intellectual capacity, health and fitness, creativity, enthusiasm, caring, flexibility, and leadership ability. Additional characteristics include: experience, professional involvement, certifications, and academic preparation. Candidates who complete the Bachelor's in Health Education with teacher certification program are expected to:

- Contribute to the promotion of behavioral changes that will enhance and maintain an optimal level of wellness for individuals and their families.

- Demonstrate a broad-based knowledge in the content areas of personal health and wellness, alcohol and drugs, communicable and non-communicable diseases, emotional health, nutrition, safety and emergency care, consumer health, and human sexuality.

- Promote healthful school living, school health services, and health education.

- Formulate and follow unit and lesson plans.

- Formulate activities and select instructional materials for health.

- Communicate effectively with other teachers, supervisors, other school personnel, and parents.

- Develop research skills and utilize a variety of methods and technologies.

- Coordinate services provided by community health service agencies (official and voluntary) at the national and local levels.

From these expectations, six distinct competencies have been identified for mastery. Table 2.2 further explains each competency area. The competency areas are:

- Content

- Instructional delivery

- Classroom management

- Personal and professional responsibility

- Planning and organization

- Pupil assessment and evaluation

Table 2.2   Competencies in Health

Competency Area	Statement of Purpose	Degree Competency
1. Content	Demonstrate competency in the field of Health Education.	Demonstrate knowledge of skills in subject matter through the ability to demonstrate a broad-base knowledge in the content area.
2. Instructional Delivery	Demonstrate competency in the field of Health Education.	Demonstrate instructional delivery skills through the ability to (1) teach lessons and (2) employ a variety of teaching methods appropriate to specific learning situations.
3. Classroom Management	Demonstrate competency in the field of Health Education.	Demonstrate classroom management and discipline skills.
4. Personal and Professional Responsibility	Demonstrate competency in the field of Health Education	Demonstrate personal and professional responsibility through the ability to (1) work with other teachers and professionals to coordinate efforts and make joint program decisions and (2) communicate effectively and work cooperatively with students, parents, teachers, and administrators
5. Planning and Organization	Demonstrate competency in the field of Health Education.	Demonstrate planning and organization skills through the ability to (1) follow and formulate developmentally appropriate unit plans (2) select and formulate developmentally appropriate activities and instructional materials, and (3) formulate a program curriculum.
6. Pupil Assessment and Evaluation	Demonstrate competency in the field of Health Education.	Demonstrate pupil assessment and evaluation skills through the ability to (1) construct valid evaluation instruments for written testing and performance rating and (2) assess and evaluate the general health status of students.

Some states may require additional areas of study for the teacher credential outside of the major including health science and state's history or government. For institutions specific requirements, check the school's catalog and plan to enroll in the proper sequence of courses.

Several education courses must be successfully completed in order to receive teaching credentials. In addition, a health educator must complete a student internship in a public school setting. Some institutions may schedule the internship during the fifth year.

In order for your teaching-learning experience to be meaningful, the student internship is done and this is the time for you to use your very own personal strengths and how these affect the participant.

The education courses listed in Table 2.1 are typical requirements for basic teaching credentials. Some states may require additional areas of study for the teaching credential outside of the major including health science, diverse students in inclusive schools and state's history or government. Check your catalog and plan to enroll in the proper sequence of classes.

AAHPERD/AAHE STANDARDS FOR HEALTH EDUCATION PROGRAMS

Health Education Standards and Key Elements

Standard I: Candidates assess individual and community needs for health education.

Key Element A: Candidates obtain health-related data about social and cultural environments, growth and development factors, needs, and interest.

Key Element B: Candidates distinguish between behaviors that foster and those that hinder well-being.

Key Element C: Candidates determine health education needs based on observed and obtained data.

Standard II: Candidates plan effective health education programs.

Key Element A: Candidates recruit school and community representatives to support and assist in program planning.

Key Element B: Candidates develop a logical scope and sequence plan for a health education program.

Key Element C: Candidates formulate appropriate and measurable learner objectives.

Key Element D: Candidates design educational strategies consistent with specified learner objectives.

Standard III: Candidates implement health education programs.

Key Element A: Candidates analyze factors affecting the successful implementation of health education and Coordinated School Health Programs (CSHPs).

Key Element B: Candidates select resources and media best suited to implement program plans for diverse learners.

Key Element C: Candidates exhibit competence in carrying out planned programs.

Key Element D: Candidates monitor educational programs, adjusting objectives and instructional strategies as necessary.

Standard IV: Candidates evaluate the effectiveness of coordinated school health programs.

Key Element A: Candidates develop plans to assess student achievement of program objectives.

Key Element B: Candidates carry out evaluation plans.

Key Element C: Candidates interpret results of program evaluation.

Key Element D: Candidates infer implications of evaluation findings for future program planning.

Standard V: Candidates coordinate provision of health education programs and services.

Key Element A: Candidates develop a plan for coordinating health education with other components of a school health program.

Key Element B: Candidates demonstrate the dispositions and skills to facilitate cooperation among health educators, other teachers, and appropriate school staff.

Key Element C: Candidates formulate practical modes of collaboration among health educators in all settings and other school and community health professionals.

Key Element D: Candidates organize professional development programs for teachers, other school personnel, community members, and other interested individuals.

Standard VI: Candidates act as a resource person in health education.

Key Element A: Candidates utilize computerized health information retrieval systems effectively.

Key Element B: Candidates establish effective consultative relationships with those requesting assistance in solving health-related problems.

Key Element C: Candidates interpret and respond to requests for health information.

Key Element D: Candidates select effective educational resource materials for dissemination.

Standard VII: Candidates communicate health and health education needs, concerns, and resources.

Key Element A: Candidates interpret concepts, purposes, and theories of health education.

Key Element B: Candidates predict the impact of societal value systems on health education programs.

Key Element C: Candidates select a variety of communication methods and techniques in providing health information.

Key Element D: Candidates foster communication between health care providers and consumers.

Certifications and Advanced Degrees

Teacher certification is required in order to teach in the traditional 6-12 school settings. It is required that teachers obtain a valid teaching certificate in the state of employment. To become certified a teacher must complete a teacher certification program at a college or university with an accredited teacher education program. Additionally the teacher must pass a standardized examination. Some states administer a national examination such as The Praxis Series: Professional Assessments for Beginning Teachers, while some states administer a state examination; such as the Alabama Perspective Teachers Test. The examination assesses basic reading, writing, and mathematics skills that all teachers are expected to have mastered. Additional examinations to measure prospective teachers' knowledge of and skills in their major fields of study may be required. Receipt of the actual teaching certificate requires submission of an application; through the university certification officer or the State Department of Education. This process may vary by state.

Colleges and universities offer graduate degrees including the master's degree, with courses useful for health educator teachers.   The educational specialist degree, a sixth-year program is offered in health education specialization. Also, the doctorate is available in health administration.

Advanced degrees are required for college/university level teaching and may be required to advance to a higher step on the salary schedule on the 6-12 level. The educational requirements for teaching health education in nontraditional settings vary by careers. Some do not require a degree; however, some college and certifications are required. Many of the nontraditional careers require advanced degrees such as masters or doctoral degrees (Refer to Chapter 5 for additional information on certifications in health.)

NON-TEACHING CAREER OPPORTUNITIES IN HEALTH

With a rapidly changing world and work environment, it is difficult to make specific career plans for the next five years, let alone the year 2015 and beyond. However, if you research and discuss with health professionals, you will discover that from a career perspective, the health profession continues to be an excellent profession. Health occupations, even during economic hardships, continue to grow and to require workers with all types of skills, abilities and interests.

With a background in health education you have numerous avenues in selecting a fulfilling and rewarding career that can meet your personal interest. But how do you know which career is best for you? First, be versatile, not just in one specific area. Second, most likely you may change you mind about your career several times during your college years and likely several times during your working years. Again, another reason to be versatile. Also, if you are satisfied with your decision of the selected career, stay with it, if not, you may choose to seek other opportunities. The health care delivery system offers great career opportunities such as:

- More primary care physicians will be needed as the focus shifts to basic health care and preventive medicine.

- Continued interest in healthy lifestyle will present opportunities for health care educators and nutritionists.

- Technology use of patient records will demand persons with computer skills

- An aging population will require the services of all types of therapists-occupational, physical, speech and hearing.

- Technological developments will require additional biomedical equipment personnel, many of whom will work for manufactures as well as health care providers.

To learn more about the career opportunities in the health profession is to talk with professionals, visit health care facilities during career days and open house, become a volunteer or take a summer job.
Educational requirements range from on-the-job training programs and apprenticeships to advanced degrees. In most instances this means a person can drop in and out of the system as desired, or follow the traditional path from high school through college and graduate school. The vast variety of health careers are too numerous to include all of them. Selected careers have been identified for inclusion in this section.

HEALTHCARE PRACTITIONER AND TECHNICAL OCCUPATIONS

Medical Care and Treatment

Communication Disorders
Audiologist
Speech Therapist

Dentistry
Dental Hygienists
Dentist, General
Dentist, Specialist
       Oral and Maxillofacial Surgeon
       Orthodontist
       Prosthodontist

Emergency Medical
Medical Emergency Technician
Paramedic

Medicine, Physician
Family and General Practitioner
Internist, General
Surgeon, General

Nursing
Certified Nurse Midwife
Licensed Practical Nurse
Nurse Manager
Nurse Practitioner
Registered Nurse
Nurse, Specialist
       Industrial Health Nurse
       Mental Health Nurse
       Occupational Health Nurse
       Public Health Nurse
School Nurse

Pharmacy
Pharmacist

Prosthesis
Orthotist
Prosthetist

Physician and Surgeon, Specialist
    Anesthesiologist
    Bariatric Physician
    Cardiovascular Disease
    Dermatologist
    Emergency Medicine Physician
    Gastroenterologist
    Neurologist
    Obstetrician and Gynecologist
    Oncologist
    Ophthalmologist
    Orthopaedic Surgeon
    Otolaryngologist
    Pediatrician
    Podiatrist
    Plastic Surgeon
    Psychiatrist
    Rheumatologist

Health Promotion

Dietetics and Nutrition
Dietitian
Nutritionist

Geriatrics
Gerontologist

Therapeutic Treatment
Arts Therapists
    Art Therapist
    Dance Therapist
    Music Therapist

Medical Technology

Clinical Technology
Cardiovascular Technologist/Technician
Diagnostic Medical Sonographer
Echocardiograph Technician
Electroencephalograph Technician
Electroneurodiagnostic Technician
Magnetic Resonance Imaging Technologist
Mammography Technologist
Nuclear Medicine Technologist
Perfusionist
Radiation Therapy Technologist
Radiologic Technician
Renal Dialysis Technician
Respiratory Technician
Surgical Technologist

Veterinary
Veterinarian
    Public Health Veterinarian
    Vector Control Veterinarian

Vision Care
Optician
Optometrist

Therapeutic Treatment
Arts Therapist
    Art Therapist
    Dance Therapist
    Drama Therapist
    Music Therapist
Athletic Trainer
Audiologist
Chiropractor
Occupational Therapist
Nutritionist
Physical Therapist
Podiatrist/Chiropodist
Speech Therapist
Radiation Therapist
Respiratory Therapist

Science and Engineering
Biological/Research Scientist
Biomedical Engineer
Biomedical Equipment Technician

Research
Biometrician
Biostatistician
Demographer
Epidemiologist
Survey Statistician
Vital Statistician

HEALTHCARE SUPPORT OCCUPATIONS

Medical Care and Treatment

Dentistry
Dental Assistant
Dental Laboratory Technician
Denturist

Medical, Physician
Hyperalimentation Technician
Medical Equipment Preparer
Orthopaedic Technician
Surgical Technician
Surgical Technologist

Nursing
Home Health Aide
Nursing Aide, Orderly, and Attendant

Occupational Health and Safety
Environmental Scientist
    Air Pollution Engineer
    Industrial Hygienist
    Occupational Hygienist
    Product Safety Engineer
Health Inspector
    Food and Drug Inspector
    Hospital Inspector
    Nursing Home Inspector
Occupational Health/Safety Technician
Safety Director

Pharmacy
Pharmacy Aide
Pharmacy Technician

Veterinary
Veterinary Technologist/Technician

Vision Care
Opthalmic Technician

Health Promotion

Dietetics and Nutrition
Dietitian Technician

Health Education
Health Educator
    Community Health Educator
    Health Promotions Specialist
    Public Health Educator
Wellness Program Director
Worksite Health Promotion Manager

Mental Health/Counseling
Medical Social Worker
Mental Health Counselor
Pastoral Counselor
Psychiatric Social Worker
Psychologist
Rehabilitation Counselor
Psychiatric Social Worker

Therapeutic Treatment
Acupuncturist
Kinesiotherapist
Massage Therapist
Occupational Therapist Assistant
Occupational Therapist Aide
Physical Therapist Assistant
Physical Therapist Aide
Psychiatric Aide
Recreational Therapist

Medical Technology

Clinical Laboratory
Cytotechnologist
Historical Technologist
Medical Laboratory Technician
Medical/Clinical Laboratory Technologist
Nuclear Laboratory Technologist
Nuclear Medicine Technician
Phlebotomist

Health Management and Support Services

Management
Adult Day Care Administrator
Health Care Facility Administrator
Health Services Administrator
Health Unit Coordinator
Hospice Director
Laboratory Manager
Laboratory Supervisor
Medical Records Administrator
Public Health Program Manager
Rehabilitation Director
Substance Abuse Center Director

Support Services
Health Information Technician
Medical Coding Specialist
Medical Records Transcriptionist
Medical Secretary

Health Information and Communication
Health Science Librarian
Laboratory Information Systems Coordinator
Medical Illustrator
Medical/Biomedical Photographer
Medical/Health Writer
Public Relations/Marketing Specialist

Salary data provided is based on information collected from the U.S. Department of Labor, Bureau of Labor Statistics and the American Medical Association. Average salaries are based on average salaries and do not necessarily represent starting salary figures.

HEALTHCARE PRACTIONER AND TECHNICAL OCCUPATIONS

MEDICAL CARE AND TREATMENT

Communication Disorders

Audiologist
Measures hearing ability, identifies hearing disorders, provides rehabilitative services, designs hearing instruments and testing equipment, and serves as consultants to government and industry on issues concerning environmental, noise-induced hearing loss. May perform research or teach at the college/university level. Requires a master's degree or higher. Practices in private practice offices, hospitals and medical centers, clinics, public and private schools, universities, rehabilitation or speech and hearing centers, health maintenance organizations, and nursing homes. Salaries range from $47,000 to $89,000 with an average of $61,000.

Speech Therapist
Assesses and treat persons with speech, language, voice, and fluency disorders. May select alternative communication systems and teach their use. May perform research or teach in colleges/universities. Requires master's degree or higher. Practice in private practice offices, hospitals and medical centers, clinics, public and private schools, universities, rehabilitation or speech and hearing centers, health maintenance organizations, and nursing homes. Salaries range from $65,000 to $105,000 with an average of $61,000.

Dentistry

Dentist, General
Diagnoses and treats diseases, injuries, and malformations of teeth and gums and related oral structures. May treat diseases of nerve, pulp, and other dental tissues affecting vitality of teeth. Medical degree from an accredited program and licensure required. Salaries range from $69,000 to $146,000 with an average of $132.000.

Oral and Maxillofacial Surgeon
Performs surgery to treat conditions, defects, injuries, and esthetic aspects of the mouth, teeth, jaws, and face. Completion of a four-year graduate degree in dentistry and licensure is required. Medical degree from accredited program and licensure is required. Salaries range from $61,000 to $185,000 with an average of $165,000.

Orthodontist
Examines, diagnoses, and treats dental malocclusions and oral cavity anomalies. Designs and fabricates appliances to realign teeth and jaws to produce and maintain normal function and to improve appearance. Medical degree from accredited program and licensure is required. Salaries range from $81,720 to $185,000 with an average of $179,000.

Prosthodontist
Constructs oral prostheses to replace missing teeth and other oral structures to correct natural and acquired deformation of mouth and jaws; restore and maintain oral function, such as chewing and speaking; and to improve appearance. Medical degree from accredited program and licensure is required. Salaries range from $56,000 to $185,000 with an average of $159,000.

Emergency Medical

Emergency Medical Technician
Provides first-aid treatment, emergency care, and transportation for sick or injured patients. Drives specially equipped emergency vehicles, determines nature and extent of an illness or injury, and performs emergency first aid procedures. Completion of EMT training program and certification is required. Employed in hospitals, police, fire, and public service departments or are employed by rescue squad or private ambulance services. Salaries range from $18,000 to $24,000 with an average of $21,000.

Paramedic
Provides first-aid treatment, emergency care, and transportation for sick or injured patients. Drives specially equipped emergency vehicles, determines nature and extent of an illness or injury, and performs emergency first aid procedures. Completion of EMT training program and certification is required. Requires 1,000 to 1,400 hours of training, must be certified or registered as an EMT-Basic, complete an EMT paramedic training program, and pass a written and practical examination. Employed in hospitals, police, fire, and public service departments or are employed by rescue squad or private ambulance services. Salaries range from $19,000 to $27,000 with an average of $23,000.

Medicine, Physician

Family and General Practitioner
Diagnoses, treats, and helps prevent diseases and injuries that commonly occur in the general population. Medical degree from accredited program and licensure is required. Salaries range from $70,000 to $167,000 with an average of $150,000.

Internist, General
Diagnoses and provides non-surgical treatment of diseases and injuries of internal organ systems. Provides care mainly for adults who have a wide range of problems associated with the internal organs. Includes subspecialists such as cardiologists and gastroenterologists. Medical degree from accredited program and licensure is required. Salaries range from $85,000 to $167,000 with an average of $135,000.

Surgeon, General
Treats diseases, injuries, and deformities by invasive methods such as manual manipulation or by using instruments and appliances. Medical degree from accredited program and licensure is required. Salaries range from $117,000 to $192,000 with an average of $154,000.

Nursing

Certified Nurse Midwife
Provides care to women during pregnancy, manages labor, delivers the baby, cares for the newborn and mother, and provides education on nutrition, breast feeding, child care, and other information needed by the mother. These are registered nurses with a bachelor's degree and additional nurse-midwifery certification requiring approximately twelve months of training. Generally self-employed and works in clinics, hospitals, or independent birthing centers. Salaries range from $40,000 to $83,000 with an average of $57,000.

Licensed Practical Nurse
Provides personal and medical care to patients who are ill or injured and works under the direction of a physician or registered nurse. Develops care plans and provides personal care such as dressing, bathing or feeding patients; cleaning and straightening patient rooms; and keeping daily records on patient's progress and activities. Completion of a state-approved practical nursing program and passing a licensing examination are required. Works in a variety of setting including hospitals, clinics, nursing homes, private homes, or institutions. Salaries range from $26,000 to $51,000 with an average of $37,000.

Nurse Manager
Plans and implements the overall nursing procedures, policies, and services for a unit and/or shift. Must be a registered nurse with at least 7 years of clinical experience in a related field. Usually manages nurses and clinical technicians in hospitals and other medical facilities. Salaries range from $30,000 to $50,000 with an average of $40,000.

Nurse Practitioner
Provides general care and treatment to patients in consultation with a physician. Has greater autonomy and in many states can practice independently and prescribe medications. Responsibilities include taking medical history, conducting physical exams, making diagnoses, ordering and interpreting lab tests and x-rays, and implementing treatment plans. Requires registered nurse degree and completion of master's level nurse practitioner program. Practices in hospitals, clinics, community centers, public health departments, and a number of other health organizations. May specialize in a particular area of care. Salaries range from $22,000 to $81,000 with an average of $45,000.

Registered Nurse
Assesses patient health problems and needs, develops and implements nursing care plans, and maintains medical records. Administers nursing care to ill, injured, convalescent, or disabled patients. May advise patients on health maintenance and disease prevention or provide case management. Completion of a Bachelor of Science Degree in Nursing (BSN) from an accredited nursing school and passing a licensure exam are required. Practices in hospitals, homes, academics, government, business, industry, medical service, and the community at large. Salaries range from $34,000 to $83,000 with an average of $57,000.

Nurse, Specialist
Registered nurses may practice in a specific area including surgery, maternity, pediatrics, geriatrics, emergency room, intensive care, orthopedics, or psychiatry. Specialty nursing areas may require additional training or education that may include degree or doctorate degree preparation. Salaries range from $34,000 to $83,000 with an average of $57,000.

Pharmacy

Pharmacist
Dispenses drugs prescribed by physicians and other health practitioners and provides information to patients about medications and their use. May advise physicians and other health practitioners on the selection, dosage, interactions, and side effects of medications. State licensure is required. After high school, it usually takes at least 6 years of study, including college and pharmacy school to become a pharmacist. Salaries range from $68,000 to $119,000 with an average of $95,000.

Prosthesis

Orthotist
Makes and fits braces and splints (orthoses) prescribed by physicians for patients needing added support for body parts that have been weakened by injury, disease, or disorders of the nerves, muscles, or bones. Special education and training in undergraduate programs and/or apprenticeships. Salaries range from $32,000 to $66,000 with an average of $55,000.

Prosthetist
Makes and fits artificial limbs (prostheses) for patients with disabilities. This includes artificial legs and arms for patients who have had amputations due to conditions such as cancer, diabetes, or injury. Special education and training in undergraduate programs and/or apprenticeships is required. Practice in hospitals, inpatient rehabilitation centers, outpatient rehabilitation centers, private practice, and industrial health centers. Salaries range from $32,000 to $66,000 with an average of $55,000.

Veterinary Science

Veterinarian
Veterinarians care for the health of pets, livestock, and/or wild animals. Diagnoses and treats animal health problems and injuries; administers preventive care to animals; and advises owners about animal feeding, behavior, and breeding. Doctor of Veterinary Medicine degree from a 4-year program at an accredited college of veterinary medicine and licensure is required. Often employed with physicians and scientists to research ways to prevent and treat various human health problems. Practices in private medical practices, zoos, aquariums, racetracks, and research laboratories. Salaries range from $44,000 to $133,000 with an average salary of $72,000.

Vision Care

Optician
Designs, measures, fits, and adapts lenses and frames for clients according to written optical prescription or specification. Measures customers for size of eyeglasses and coordinates frames with facial and eye measurements and optical prescription. Prepares work orders for optical laboratories containing instructions for grinding and mounting lenses in frames. Includes contact lens opticians. Must hold an associate opticinary degree or apprenticeship for a required number of hours. Most states require licensure and the passing of a national and state board examination. Certain states require passing an additional national examination to fit and dispense contact lenses. Salaries range from $24,000 to $48,000 with an average of $32,000.

Optometrist
Diagnoses, manages, and treats conditions and diseases of the human eye and visual system. Examines eyes and visual system, diagnoses problems or impairments, prescribes corrective lenses, and provides treatment. Completion of accredited 4-year optometry program and passing a written and clinical state board examination is required. May prescribe therapeutic drugs to treat specific eye conditions. Salaries range from $45,000 to $166,000 with an average of $135,000.

HEALTH PROMOTION

Dietetics and Nutrition

Clinical Dietician
Assesses nutritional needs of patients; plans menus and meals based on an individual's dietary needs, restrictions, and nutritional requirements; instructs patients on proper nutrition and diet, and consults with physicians and other health care professionals to assess the needs of patients. Bachelor's degree with a major in dietetics, nutrition, food service systems management, or related filed is required. Practices in hospitals, clinics, nursing homes, health maintenance organizations, government departments, home health care agencies, and public health organizations. Salaries range from $16,000 to $38,000 with an average salary of $26,000.

Nutritionist

Assesses nutritional problems in individuals and population groups, develops and implements programs to change patterns of food consumption and weight control, and conducts fundamental research into human and animal nutrition. Practices in government and private agencies, institutions, and industries. A master's degree or Ph.D., state licensing, and board certification are required. Salaries range from $25,000 to $60,000 with an average of $40,000.

Geriatrics

Gerontologist

Specializes in working with and educating elderly patients. Studies the physical, mental, and social changes that occur with the aging process in older people and how they fit into society. Research gerontologists conduct research on the aging process and the living environments of the elderly. Applied gerontologists work directly with the elderly, communicating with and analyzing individuals, families, and groups. Administrative gerontologists develop programs and coordinate services. Practices in nursing homes, senior citizen centers, and other similar facilities. May have degrees or training in nursing, psychology, sociology, or other social services-related professions. Salaries range dependent upon area of work education and experiences. Salaries range from $29,000 to $55,000 with an average of $41,800.

Therapeutic Treatment

Arts Therapist

Plans, organizes, and directs medically approved programs as part of the care and treatment of patients of all ages who suffer from physical, mental, or emotional illnesses. Utilizes an art form: art, dance, music, or drama and other techniques such as counseling, behavior modification, and physical activity to achieve patient therapeutic goals. Helps patients build confidence and self-esteem and deals with pain or trauma and manage stress by facilitating expression of feelings in positive and effective ways. Knowledge of a variety of psychotherapeutic, physical rehabilitation, teaching techniques, and the art form are required. Practices in a variety of settings such as hospitals, schools, mental health centers, prisons, and businesses. Salaries range from $23,000 to $135,000 with an average of $44,000.

Athletic Trainer

Specializes in preventing, recognizing, managing, and rehabilitating injuries that result from physical activity. Practices under the direction of a licensed physician and in cooperation with other health care professionals, athletics administrators, coaches, and parents as part of a health care team. Requires a minimum of a bachelor's degree from an accredited athletic training program and passing a national certification exam. Ongoing continuing education requirements to remain certified. Salaries range from $22,000 to $59,000 with an average of $39,000.

Chiropractor

Promotes correct physical alignment to maintain health without drugs and surgery. Adjusts spinal column and other articulations of the body to correct abnormalities of the human body believed to be caused by interference with the nervous system. Examines patients to determine nature and extent of disorders. May utilize supplementary measures such as exercise, rest, water, light, heat, and nutritional therapy. Doctor of Chiropractic degree and national and state licensure required. Salaries range from $46,000 to $96,000 with an average of $65,000.

Occupational Therapist

Assesses, plans, organizes, and participates in rehabilitative programs that help restore vocational, homemaking, and daily living skills, as well as general independence to disabled persons suffering from mental, physical, developmental or emotional conditions. A master's degree or higher in occupational therapy from an accredited educational program and passing a national certification examination is the minimum requirement. Practices in rehabilitation centers, hospitals, private homes and other health care and community settings. Salaries range from $41,000 to $89,000 with an average of $60,000.

Physical Therapist

Assesses, plans, organizes, and participates in rehabilitative programs that improve mobility, relieve pain, increase strength, and decrease or prevent deformity of patients suffering from disease or injury to restore, maintain, and promote overall fitness and health. Master's or doctoral degree and licensure are required. Practices in hospitals, clinics, private offices, homes, and schools. Salaries range from $47,000 to $95,000 with an average of $66,000.

MEDICAL TECHNOLOGY

Clinical Technology

Diagnostic Medical Sonographer
Uses waves to generate images for assessment and diagnosis of various medical conditions and is most commonly associated with obstetrics and pregnancy. Practices as a contract employee in health care facilities and mobile imaging services. Completion of a 1-4 year training program in required. Annual certification examinations are required. Salaries range from $24,000 to $38,000 with an average of $32,000.

Echocardiograph Technician
Performs electrocardiographs according to established policies and procedures. Requires a high school diploma and is a graduate of an accredited EKG program with 0-2 years of clinical experience. Salaries range from $18,000 to $30,000 with an average of $24,000.

Mammography Technologist
Operates X-ray equipment and performs various mammography related procedures. Prepares and maintains records and files and cleans and makes minor adjustments to equipment as needed. Requires completion of a formal radiologic technology training program from an accredited program and certification in Diagnostic Mammography. Practices in hospitals, clinics, and other health facilities. Salaries range from $46,000 to $63,000 with an average of $54,000.

Magnetic Resonance Imaging Technologist
Operates magnetic resonance imaging equipment to produce cross-sectional images of the body for the purpose of diagnosis of disease and injury. Associate's degree in Radiologic Technology program with MRI as a post primary certification or equivalent from a two-year college or technical school and passing a national certification examination is required. Practice in hospitals, clinics, and other health facilities. Salaries range from $56,000 to $77,000 with an average of $62,000.

Perfusionist
Operates heart-lung machines and monitors the circulatory and physiological processes during surgery. Requires a bachelor's degree in science, nursing, or other program requiring significant science coursework. Some programs prefer students with prior training or coursework in medical technology, respiratory care, anatomy, physiology, chemistry, or pharmacology. Practices in hospitals, surgical practices, and group practices. Salaries range from $58,000 to $100,000 with an average of $70,000.

Radiologic Technologists and Technicians
Uses X-ray machines, ultrasound machines, magnetic resonance scanners, positron emission scanners, and other technologically advanced machines to help diagnose and treat illnesses and injuries under the direction of a physician. Explains procedures and prepares patients for radiological tests and treatments, makes radiologic images, and maintains equipment. Completion of two-year radiologic technology training program is required. Practices in hospitals, clinics, medical laboratories, nursing homes, and in private industry. Salaries range from $44,000 to $92,000 with an average of $66,000.

Radiation Therapist
Provides radiation therapy to patients as prescribed by a radiologist. Duties may include reviewing prescriptions and diagnoses; acting as a liaison with physicians and supportive care personnel; and preparing equipment and maintaining records, reports, and files. May assist in dosimetry procedures and tumor localization. Bachelor's degree, associate's degree, and certificate in radiation therapy generally are required. Some states, as well as many employers, require that radiation therapists be certified. Practices in hospitals or cancer treatment centers. Salaries range from $45,000 to $92,000 with an average of $66,000.

Research

Biostatistician
Helps anticipate needs and improves decision making with regard to health problems, programs, and technologies through the development and operation of ongoing statistical information systems concerned with vital events, health statuses, and program operations. Helps with the proper design and carrying out of studies and the analysis and interpretation of data obtained from such studies. In local and state agencies employment includes the collection, tabulation, and analysis of statistics bearing on all aspects of health problems and programs. In state, provincial, federal, and academic settings employment includes providing assistance to investigators in the design, performance, and data analysis of research on health problems and programs. In academic institutions employment includes training health workers in the use and interpretation of statistics and carrying out research to discover improved ways of using statistical measures and procedures. Salaries range from $35,000 to $60,000 with am average salary pf $45,000.

Epidemiologist
Determines disease frequencies and trends in populations and factors that increase or reduce disease and disability. Employed in the design and execution of studies or information systems concerned with ascertaining distribution and determinants of disease or disability. In academic settings epidemiologists teach, research, and assist clinical investigators in the study of disease and evaluation of new or improved measures for disease prevention, therapy, and rehabilitation. A master's degree is preferred. Salaries range from $40,000 to $60,000 with an average of $50,000.

HEALTHCARE SUPPORT OCCUPATIONS

Medical Care and Treatment

Dentistry

Dental Assistant
Provides support functions for dentists including assisting with dental procedures and laboratory work, including dental radiography support and functions. Completing a dental-assisting training program is not required. May require passing written and/or practical exam. Passing national and state examinations required for performing specialized duties such as radiological procedures. Practices in general or specialty dental offices with some opportunity to work for dental laboratories, hospitals, and insurance companies. Certification is required. Salaries range from $22,000 to $43,000 with an average of $30,000.

Dental Hygienist
Cleans calcareous deposits, accretions, and stains from teeth and beneath the margins of the gums using dental instruments. Feels lymph nodes under patient's chin to detect swelling or tenderness that could indicate presence of oral cancer. Feels and visually examines gums for sores and signs of disease. May conduct dental health clinics for community groups to augment services of a dentist. May require an associate's degree or its equivalent and 2-4 years of experience and is licensed as a dental hygienist. Salaries range from $15,000 to $20,000 with an average of $18,000.

Dental Laboratory Technician
Constructs models and casts of teeth to make dentures, bridgework, or other dental prosthetics. Completing dental laboratory technology program is not required. Practices in private dental laboratories, dentist's offices, hospitals, or dental suppliers. Salaries range from $15,000 to $22,000 with an average of $18,000.

Denturist
Constructs and fits removable oral prostheses. Completion of accredited course, usually 2-3 years in length, in addition to having at least four years experience and background in dental technology and certification required. Salaries range from $21,000 to $43,000 with an average of $30,000.

Medical, Physician

Hyperalimentation Technician
Provides nutritional and vitamin related prescription drugs and medications to patients and prepares special intravenous solutions. Counsels patients and family on use of various medications. Updates and maintains supplies to identify and reorder outdated stock and ensure that stock is maintained in accordance with manufacturer's requirements. May require an associate's degree or its equivalent with 2-4 years of experience in the field or in a related area. Salaries range from $27,000 to $34,000 with an average of $32,000.

Medical Assistant
Performs administrative and clinical tasks under supervision of physicians and other licensed health practitioners. Responsibilities and salaries are dependent upon the practitioner's specialty, location and size of the practice, qualifications, responsibilities, and experience. Salaries range from $16,460 to $74,390 with an average of $28,000.

Medical Equipment Preparer
Prepares, sterilizes, installs, cleans, delivers, sets up, operates, and inspects surgical instruments and medical equipment. No advanced training required. Salaries range from $19,000 to $37,000 with an average of $26,000.

Surgical Assistant/Operating Room Technician
Assists surgical team during operative procedures by arranging and inventorying sterile set-up for operations. Assists in preparing and moving patients and in cleaning the operating theatre. Completion of accredited operating room technician program, certification, and 2-4 years of experience required. Salary range varies with experience. Salaries range from $20,000 to $40,000 with an average of $30,000.

Physician Assistant
Provides healthcare services typically performed by a physician, under the supervision of a physician. Conducts complete physicals, provides treatment, and counsels patients. In some cases may prescribe medication. Must graduate from an accredited education program for physician assistants. Salaries range from $43,000 to $92,000 with an average of $75,000.

Nursing

Home Health Aide
Provides and supports patients with personal care. Requires a high school diploma or its equivalent and 0-2 years of experience in the field or in a related area. May be expected to meet certain state certifications and be CPR certified. Usually reports to a registered nurse. Salary ranges between $15,000 and $20,000 with an average of $18,000.

Nursing Aide, Orderly, and Attendant
Provides basic patient care under direction of nursing staff. Performs duties such as feeding, bathing, dressing, grooming, moving patients, or changing linens. On the job training. Salary range between $16,000 to $31,000 with an average of $23,000.

Occupational Health and Safety

Environmental Scientist
Performs laboratory and field tests to monitor the environment and investigates sources of pollution, including those that affect health. Under direction of an environmental scientist or specialist, may collect samples of gasses, soil, water, and other materials for testing and take corrective actions as assigned. Educational background usually includes disciplinary training in one or more of the natural sciences plus advanced courses in those aspects of environmental health relevant to their primary discipline. Employment is available at all levels of government, public and private organizations, and industry to provide technical knowledge and methods in the investigation, planning, controlling, and regulation of matters pertaining to environmental health hazards. Salaries range from $24,000 to $61,000 with an average of $38,000.

Health Inspector
Conducts investigations of work environments to determine if safety and health requirements are being met. Bachelor's degree and 2-4 years of experience in the field or in a related area is required. Salaries range from $30,000 and $50,000 with an average of $40,000.

Occupational Health/Safety Technician
Reviews, evaluates, and analyzes work environments and designs programs and procedures to control, eliminate, and prevent disease or injury caused by chemical, physical, biological agents, or ergonomic factors. Conducts inspections and enforces adherence to laws and regulations governing the health and safety of individuals. May be employed in the public or private sector. Includes environmental protection officers. Salaries range from $35,000 to $87,000 with an average of $58,000.

Occupational Hygienist
Responsible for anticipating, recognizing, evaluating, controlling, and preventing health hazards in the working environment with the goal of protecting the health and well-being of workers and the community through the assessment and control of chemical, physical, or biological hazards that could cause disease or discomfort. Position may require the individual to communicate hazard, risk, and appropriate protective procedures; to evaluate and occasionally to design ventilation systems; and to manage people and programs for the preservation of health and well-being of those who enter the workplace. Bachelor's degree from an accredited college or university in industrial hygiene, physical science or life science is required. Salaries range from $57,000 to $82,000 with an average of $69,000.

Safety Director
Directs an organization's safety programs. Develops, implements, and manages safety programs, procedures, and policies. Responsible for maintenance of safety/accident records. May require a bachelor's degree and 10-12 years of experience. Salaries range from $25,000 to $40,000 with an average of $32,000.

Pharmacy

Pharmacy Aide
Records drugs delivered to the pharmacy, stores incoming merchandise, and informs the supervisor of stock needs. May operate cash register and accept prescriptions for filling. On-the-job training. Salaries range from $14,000 to $30,000 with an average of $19,000.

Pharmacy Technician
Helps licensed pharmacists provide medication and other health care products to patients. Receives and verifies prescriptions; prepares medication for clients through mixing, counting pills and labeling bottles; prices and fills prescriptions; obtains approval from the pharmacist; fills out patient paperwork and insurance claims; inventories and stocks medications; and performs administrative duties such as answering phones, stocking shelves, and operating cash registers. Completion of accredited training program and certification is recommended. Employed in hospitals, drug store pharmacies, nursing homes, and other health care facilities. Salaries range from $18,000 to $37,000 with an average of $27,000.

Veterinary Science

Veterinary Technologist/Technician
Performs medical tests in a laboratory environment for use in the treatment and diagnosis of diseases in animals. Prepares vaccines and serums for prevention of diseases. Prepares tissue samples, takes blood samples, administers laboratory tests, cleans and sterilizes instruments and materials and maintains equipment and machines. Associate's degree from accredited program in veterinary technology and certification is required. Salaries range from $18,000 to $39,000 with an average salary of $27,000.

Health Promotion

Dietetics and Nutrition

Dietetic Technician
Practices under the supervision of dietitians and assists in planning menus and educating individuals on proper nutrition. Employed in cafeterias or kitchens in health care settings such as hospitals, clinics, nursing homes, health maintenance organizations, government departments, home health care agencies, and public health organizations. As associate's degree from a dietetic technician program is required. Salaries range from $17,000 to $24,000 with an average of $28,000.

Geriatrics

Geriatric Nurse Assistant
Performs a variety of duties to help care for older patients under the supervision of nurses and physicians. Geriatric care providers of all types work in a variety of settings, including community organizations, retirement communities, academic settings, health care and long-term organizations, government agencies, and professional organizations. On-the-job training. Salaries range from $12,000 to $24,000 with an average salary of $18,000.

Health Education

Health Educator
Promotes, maintains, and improves individual and community health by assisting individuals and communities to adopt healthy behaviors. Collects and analyzes data to identify community needs prior to planning, implementing, monitoring, and evaluating programs designed to encourage healthy lifestyles, policies and environments. May also serve as a resource to assist individuals, other professionals, or the community. May administer fiscal resources for health education programs. Practices in health education and health promotion programs in schools, companies, clinical, and other community settings. Salaries range from $25,000 to $72,000 with an average of $41,000.

Mental Health/Counseling

Mental Health Technician
Establishes a therapeutic relationship with assigned patients and helps patients with daily living and overall maintenance of a therapeutic environment in the psychiatric unit. Takes vital signs, weighs patients, and collects routine specimens. Requires a high school diploma or its equivalent and 0-2 years of related experience. Salaries range from $15,000 to $22,000 with an average of $18,000.

Mental Health Counselor
Counsels families, individuals, couples, and groups to promote optimum mental health and well-being. Helps individuals address marital problems, stress management, substance abuse, addictions, parenting problems, family problems, suicidal ideation, self-esteem, aging problems, emotional issues, and mental health issues. Many counselors work in hospitals, clinics, counseling centers, government agencies, corporations, youth homes, and private practices. Works closely with other mental health professionals, such as psychiatrists, psychologists, social workers, school counselors, marriage and family therapists, and psychiatric nurses. Master's degree in mental health counseling or related specialization, two years of supervised post-master's clinical experience, and licensure are required. Continuing education required every two years for license renewal. Salaries range from $24,000 to $62,000 with an average of $38,000.

Medical and Public Health Social Worker
Provides individuals, families, or vulnerable populations with the psychosocial support needed to cope with chronic, acute, or terminal illnesses, such as Alzheimer's, cancer, or AIDS. Assures patients' medically related emotional and social needs are met and maintained throughout medical treatment. Advises family care givers, provides patient education and counseling, and makes referrals for other social services. Works in multi-disciplinary settings with other health and human service professionals in hospitals, outpatient medical facilities, hospices, rehabilitation facilities, physician group practices, skilled nursing facilities, nursing homes, and home health agencies. Bachelor's degree or higher in social work or a closely related field is required. Other licensure and certifications may be required based on area of employment. Salaries range from $48,000 to $64,000 with an average of $53,000.

Therapeutic Treatment

Acupuncturist
Uses technique of traditional Chinese medicine in which metal needles are inserted into the skin at specially designated points for treatment of pain and various other ailments. Licensure is required. Salaries range from $43,000 to $59,000 with an average of $53,000.

Kinesiotherapist
Applies scientifically based exercise principles to enhance strength, endurance, and mobility of individuals with functional limitations or requiring extended physical conditioning. Determines and administers appropriate musculoskeletal, neurological, ergonomic, biomechanical, psychosocial, and task-specific functional tests and measures. Establishes goal-specific treatment plan in collaboration with the client to restore, maintain, and improve overall functional abilities. Bachelor's degree in kinesiotherapy or related field and certification are required. Employed in medical centers, public and private hospitals, sports medicine facilities, rehabilitation facilities, learning disability centers, schools, colleges and universities, private practice, and as exercise consultants. Salaries range from $30,000 to $60,000 with an average of $48,000.

Massage Therapist
Performs massage therapy techniques to control pain, reduce stress, and promote relaxation. May require a high school diploma or equivalent and requires certification as a massage therapist. Employed in private practice, health and wellness center, hotel, resort, physical therapy center, rehabilitation clinic, hospital, sports organization, spa, cruise ship, or are self-employed. Salaries range from $33,000 to $60,000 with an average of $48,000.

Occupational Therapist Aide
Performs delegated, selected, or routine tasks in specific situations under close supervision of an occupational therapist or occupational therapy assistant. Salaries range from $17,000 to $44,000 with an average of $25,000.

Physical Therapist Assistant
Performs a variety of tasks under the direction and supervision of physical therapists including exercises, massages, electrical stimulation, paraffin baths, hot and cold packs, traction, and ultrasound. Records and reports patient's responses to treatment. Associate degree from an accredited physical therapist assistant program and state licensure required. Salaries range from $26,000 to $57,000 with an average of $41,000.

Physical Therapist Aide
Performs a variety of tasks under the direction and supervision of physical therapists or physical therapist assistants. High school diploma required. On-the-job training. Salaries range from $15,000 to $36,000 with an average of $21,000.

Recreational Therapist
Plans, directs, and coordinates medically-approved recreation programs for patients in hospitals, nursing homes, or other institutions. Activities include sports, trips, dramatics, social activities, and arts and crafts. Assesses patient condition and recommends appropriate recreational activity. Bachelor's degree and licensure are required. Salaries range from $21,000 to $56,000 with an average of $35,000.

Medical Technology

Clinical Laboratory

Cytotechnologist
Prepares microscopic slides of cells of the human body to detect cell abnormalities under the supervision of a pathologist. Studies the structure and function of the human body's cells in the diagnosis of cancer. Bachelor's degree and certification required. Practices in hospitals, clinics, or private laboratories. May also teach or do research. Salaries range from $22,000 to $50,000 with an average of $32,000.

Histologic Technologist
Prepares microscopic slides from tissue samples for examination by pathologists and scientists. Also know as histotechnologists or tissue technologists. Requires a bachelor's degree with a major in medical technology or life sciences. Certification may be required. Practices in the pathology laboratory of a hospital or clinic or a medical or research laboratory. Salaries range from $22,000 to $51,000 with an average of $32,000.

Phlebotomist
Draws and collects blood samples from patients or blood donors for medical tests and/or blood donations. Verifies records and prepares specimens for laboratory analysis. Requires a high school diploma and/or certification by a nationally recognized body and 0-3 years of related experience. Practices in hospital laboratories, private laboratories, clinics, large medical offices, and blood banks. Salaries range from $18,000 to $40,000 with an average of $27,000.

Health Management and Support Services

Management

Adult Day Care Administrator
Identifies health, education, and psychosocial needs of older individuals in the community and develops programs and activities for those that do not live in a long-term care or retirement facility. Requires a bachelor's degree with at least 7 years of experience in the field. Salaries range from $20,000 to $40,000 with an average of $30,000.

Health Services Administrator
Plans, implements, manages, coordinates, and evaluates programs for the delivery of health care for the aging. Designs administrative systems appropriate for the needs of the population being serviced. Employed at all levels of government and in the private sector. Bachelor's degree or administrative experience without other advanced training is required. Salaries range from $30,000 to $50,000 with an average of $40,000.

Hospice Director
Directs, supervises, and governs the hospice program including in-patient care, home care and bereavement follow-up. Requires a bachelor's degree in nursing with at least 7 years of experience in the field. Salaries range from $25,000 to $50,000 with an average of $32,000.

Medical Records Administrator
Coordinates personnel that handle permanent medical records of patients by analyzing, coding, indexing and storing records. Ensures records are accurate, complete, and adhere to standards. Associate's degree or equivalent with 2-4 years of experience in the field or in a related area required. Salaries range from $38,000 to $81,000 with an average of $58,000.

Wellness Program Administrator
Assists in the administration of wellness programs and activities designed to improve employee health and well-being. Responsible for recommending changes and/or additions to programs that reflect the needs of the employees. May require a bachelor's degree in the area of specialty and 2-4 years of experience in the field or in a related area. Salaries range from $32,000 to $62,000 with an average of $47,000.

Rehabilitation Director
Directs the programs and staff of the rehabilitation services department. Sets and implements guidelines for rehabilitation programs. May require an advanced degree and professional certification with at least 7 years of direct experience in the field. Salaries range from $30,000 to $60,000 with an average of $45,000.

Substance Abuse Center Director
Directs the clinical, managerial, and administrative aspects of substance abuse programs. Evaluates treatment procedures to ensure attainment of objectives and goals regarding rehabilitation from drug/alcohol dependency. Employed with community agencies and programs to ensure continuity in the type and level of patient care. Requires a bachelor's degree and at least 7 years of experience in the field or in a related field. Salaries range from $30,000 to $50,000 with an average if $40,000.

Support Services

Health Information Technician
Organizes, evaluates, and records patient health information for completeness and accuracy. Ensures all forms are completed and properly identified and signed, and all necessary information is in the computer. Completion of accredited record technicians course and passing a written examination is required. Employed by hospitals, physician's offices, clinics, nursing homes, and home health agencies. Median salary ranges from $20,000 to $44,000 with an average of $30,000 for accredited health information technicians.

Medical Records Transcriptionist
Transcribes and edits prerecorded medical dictation into hard copies of patient's assessments, diagnostics, therapies, and other medical reports. Completion of accredited medical transcription program, experience in acute care, and a passing score on national certification examination are required. Employed in hospitals, offices, clinics, laboratories, medical libraries, transcription offices or at home. Salaries range from $22,000 to $33,000 with an average of $28,000.

Health Information and Communication

Medical Librarian
Provides assistance in computer searches, inter-library loans, cataloging, reference, acquisitions, circulation, and system development and maintenance. Offers library instruction and education programs for library patrons. Position may require a bachelor's degree in area of specialty and 2-4 years of experience in the field or in a related area. Salary range varies according to experience.

Medical Illustrator
Creates graphic representations of medical or biological subjects for use in textbooks, pamphlets, exhibits, instructional films, civil/criminal legal procedures, and teaching models. Uses most current technology and graphic design software to describe and illustrate medical concepts and processes. May specialize in certain anatomical areas such as the brain or heart. Bachelor's degree combining art and premedical courses is required. Employed in medical schools, hospitals, research organizations, publishing companies, advertising agencies, pharmaceutical manufacturers, or large medical centers with teaching and research programs. Many work as free-lance artists and contract out services. Salaries range from $33,000 to $66,000 with an average of $42,000.

Medical/Biomedical Photographer
Uses photography to document scientific information that relates to biology, chemistry, medicine, and other health-related subjects for textbooks, pamphlets, exhibits, instructional films, civil/criminal legal procedures, and teaching models. May document surgical procedures and record patient's medical progress over time or autopsy. Associate or bachelor's degree, photography experience and certification required. Employed in medical schools, hospitals, research organizations, publishing companies, advertising agencies, pharmaceutical manufacturers, or large medical centers with teaching and research programs. Salaries range form $31,000 to $47,000 with an average of $38,000.

Medical/Health Writer
Analyzes and interprets health related issues for use by other professionals and the general public in professional journals, newspaper health columns, television and radio broadcasts, brochures, textbooks, and instructional manuals. Bachelor's degree with major/minor in science, English, or journalism and certification is required. Employed by publishing companies, pharmaceutical companies, advertising agencies, educational institutions, hospitals, government agencies, radio and television stations, and medical equipment companies. Salaries range from $41,000 to $71,000 with an average of $55,000.

THE FUTURE OF HEALTH CAREERS

One of the most dynamic and fastest growing areas of employment in the United States today is the field of medical careers. Exponential growth is expected to occur between the years 2002 and 2012 with an increase of approximately thirty percent or 4.3 million jobs for all areas of the medical industry over the next eight years.

Healthcare worker shortages are well documented with more than one million practitioner openings available today. There are many potential job opportunities with over 200 different careers in the healthcare field. The demand for health professionals will continue to increase dramatically as the use of technology accelerates and the population continues to live longer.

Health professionals provide care for millions of people everyday and the demand for health professionals is rapidly increasing. This increase brings with it a wide range of opportunities and challenges. Individuals are becoming more aware of general health and health issues and showing more concern for their own personal health. Individuals are living longer and the nation's largest population, the "baby boomers," is now reaching retirement age. Also, individuals are considering alternative methods of treating and preventing illnesses and promoting wellness.

Now, more than ever, if you want a career where you can make a real difference in people's lives and make the world a better place – the health field is for you. There are literally hundreds of rewarding careers in medicine and healthcare. One of them could be waiting for you.

SUMMARY

The process of preparing for a career is systematic – you make a career decision based on a series of interests, skills and experiences developed over a period of time. For the future, the definition of health encompasses a sense of individual and social responsibility. Healthy people are concerned about others and the greater environment rather than on one's own personal health. There is a vast difference in health status between various social groups and actively promoting community actions to erase disparities. In preparing for your life's work, it a good choice to explore the possibilities of a career in the health profession. This decision may lead to successful job performance and job satisfaction in the fast-growing health industry.

REFLECTIONS

1. Compare and contrast the four categories of health: health education, health promotion, community health and population health. Use Laboratory Activity 2.1 for your response.

2. Using the research data from Laboratory Activity 2.2, determine the advantages and disadvantages of a selected health career and explain why you would or would not choose that particular career.

3. Review the six competencies in health in this chapter. Reflect on your coursework and practical experiences to determine your level of proficiency in each area.

WEB SITES

www.aahperd.org/aahe/
American Association for Health Education

www.acha.org
American College Health Association

www.eatright.org
American Dietetic Association

www.americanheart.org/
American Heart Association

www.aota.org
American Occupational Therapy Association

www.apha.org
American Public Health Association

www.apta.org
American Physical Therapy Association

www.cdc.gov
Centers for Disease Control and Prevention

www.healthcareers.net
Health Careers

www.studentdoc.com/medical-careers.html
Medical Careers

www.medicalcareerinfo.com
Medical Career Information

www.nche.org
National Center for Health Education

www.onhealth.com
On Health.com

www.fastcompany.salary.com
Salary.com health career descriptions with the salary ranges

www.learningandlife.com/healthcare-careers/top-medical-careers.php
Top Growth Medical Careers

www.who.org
World Health Organization

www.womenshealthalliance.com/
Women's Health Alliance – women's health issues

BIBLIOGRAPHY

Anspaugh, David J. and Ezell, Gene. (2007). *Teaching Today's Health,* 8th ed. Boston: MA, Pearson Education.

Floyd, P., Mimms, S., and Yelding, C. (2008). *Personal Health: Perspectives and Lifestyles*, 4th ed. Belmont: CA, Wadsworth/Thomson.

Joint Committee on Health Education Terminology. (1991). Report of the 1990 joint committee on health education terminology. *Journal of Health Education.* 22: 97-108.

LABORATORY ACTIVITY 2.1

NAME _____ DATE _____

COURSE _____ SECTION _____

Research the four categories of health on the Internet. Compare and contrast the categories. Enter you findings in the table below. Discuss your results with the class.

Category	Comparisons	Contrasts
Health Education		
Health Promotion		
Community Health		
Population Health		

LABORATORY ACTIVITY 2.2

NAME _____ DATE _____

COURSE _____ SECTION _____

Interview an individual in three health career areas to determine their opinion of the advantages and disadvantages of the career. Record your findings below.

CHAPTER 3

INTRODUCTION TO CAREERS IN PHYSICAL EDUCATION

"The vigor of our citizens is one of America's most precious resources. If we waste and neglect this resource, if we allow it to swindle and grow soft then we will destroy much of our ability to meet the great and vital challenges that confront our people. We will be unable to realize our full potential as a nation."

John F. Kennedy

KEY CONCEPTS

1. The purpose of physical education is to improve quality of life through physical activity.
2. A variety of trends contribute to past and future changes in physical education.
3. There are advantages and disadvantages to teaching physical education.
4. The individual must have the appropriate educational and practical experiences to teach physical education.
5. Students who complete a basic teacher certification program in physical education are expected to demonstrate six distinct competencies.
6. There are many diverse careers in physical education.

INTRODUCTION

Career opportunities in physical education have become progressively more diverse and have expanded tremendously over the past thirty years. A wide variety of careers ranging from Physical Education teacher, to researcher, to administrator and many more in between are available. Physical educators who are open-minded and have drive, creativity, and a strong work ethic have numerous open avenues to select a fulfilling and rewarding career that will meet personal and professional interests. Directing your career toward any one of these many areas could create a new and satisfying career opportunity for you.

Figure 3.1 Physical Education and Related Careers

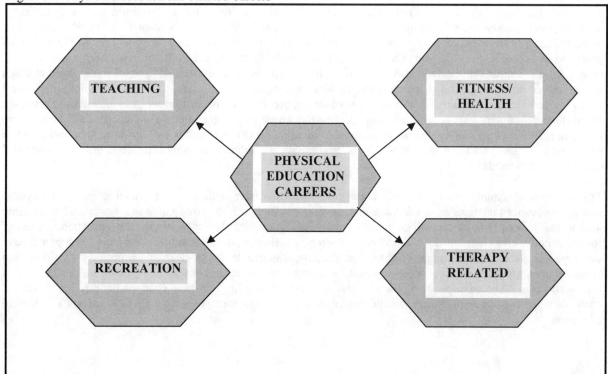

What is Physical Education?

Physical education is many things to many people. Traditionally, physical education was defined as formal instruction in physical activities that took place in schools and colleges/universities. Physical education programs focused on teaching sports and games to able-bodied school-aged children. Today, physical education encompasses an expansive range of people and places. People of all ages and abilities participate in physical education not only in schools and colleges/universities; but also in the workplace, in the community, in hospitals, in commercial gyms, in nursing homes, in resorts, and even in the home and other places.

Physical education engages individuals in movement experiences that contribute to their total growth and development. Physical education programs help individuals achieve movement competence, develop and maintain physical fitness, learn personal health and wellness skills, apply movement concepts, develop lifelong activity skills, and demonstrate positive social skills. The purpose of physical education is to improve the quality of life of those who participate. Physical activity, fitness, health and wellness are improved through physical education. All movement that contributes to improved health is physical activity. Those movements that improve heart and other bodily functions through endurance and resistive exercises develop physical fitness. Health is the well-being of the body and includes disease and illness. Wellness consists of the physical, mental, spiritual, and emotional aspects that facilitate healthy behaviors.

CAREER OPPORTUNITIES IN PHYSICAL EDUCATION

Prior to the 1970s, physical education professionals were positioned in roles of physical education teacher and/or coach. With the changes in society, demographics, trends in the discipline and advocacy, physical education has changed dramatically. Societal trends have contributed to changes in the discipline of physical education and ensuing careers. Technological advancements and other changes have resulted in more leisure time and larger discretionary incomes for many people. In addition to having more leisure time and more money, people are living longer and healthier lives due to modern medicine. Many of these individuals are choosing to spend much of their extra time in fitness and recreational activities.

The demographics of the United States are changing. People are living longer and birth rates are declining, increasing the average age of the population. It is expected that 18.5% of the population will be 65 years old or older in 2025. There is an increasing number of very elderly people. It is projected that 7 million people will be 85 years old and older in 2025, up from 3.8 million in 1996. In 2020, an estimated 25% of the elderly population will be minorities. Cultural diversity is also on the rise. It is likely that in 2020 over 45% of all school aged children will be ethnic minorities. The changing demographics have significant implications for the discipline of physical education and available careers. Quality physical education programs are needed for the growing elderly population for health enhancement and recreational pursuits. Programs must be designed to take into account and be sensitive to the needs of an increasingly diverse population. Providing access to physical activity through school physical education programs is not enough. More diverse and innovative approaches to meeting these growing needs will continue to be expanded.

Trends in the discipline of physical education have affected career options. The scientific study of physical education advanced its status as an academic discipline. As a discipline, the propagation of research and scholarship lead to the development of specialized areas of study and broadened the scope of physical education. Areas of specialization such as kinesiology, biomechanics, exercise physiology, motor learning, and motor development have developed. Research has also spawned changes in the American people. It has clearly documented the link between health, fitness, and total well-being. As a result, Americans are adopting a new attitude about health, fitness, and total well-being. The concepts of physical fitness and movement education have changed the physical education curriculum and, along with research, have contributed the development of a host of new careers in physical education.

Advocacy has evolved from the research in physical education. The health-related benefits of physical activity have been brought to the attention of the American public. The *Surgeon General's Report on Physical Activity and Health*, the American Heart Association, the American Medical Association, the President's Council on Physical Fitness and Sports, the Governor's Commissions/Councils on Physical Fitness and Sports and other organizations strongly advocate the need for and benefits of physical education and physical activity. The research has shown unmistakable relationships between physical activity and the reductions in the severity of some disabling conditions and increases in the occurrence of chronic diseases such as heart attack, stroke, diabetes, depression, colon cancer and osteoporosis. Americans are buying into physical education and physical activity. Individuals are initiating fitness/health programs and participating in a variety of physical activities in many settings. Employers are providing fitness and health programs for employees in an effort to help prevent excessive lost labor time and health care costs due to preventable absenteeism and illness. Advocacy has led to the creation of many new job opportunities for professionals in physical education and related careers.

The purpose of this chapter is to familiarize you with a broader scope of diverse career opportunities available in physical education. Teaching will be discussed and a thumbnail profile including responsibilities, qualifications, and general salary range for selected related physical education careers will be presented. The selected related careers are in the areas of fitness/health, recreation, and therapy. Additionally, careers in related associations/organizations are profiled.

By no means is this list inclusive of all career opportunities available in the field physical education. By examining the various options in physical education careers you can determine which choice is best suited to your interests, aptitudes and experiences. Hopefully, it will assist you in making a professional choice that will lead you to the achievement of a rewarding professional life in the field of physical education.

TEACHING PHYSICAL EDUCATION

Careers in the teaching profession appear to be promising. Education, health, and business services are predicted to provide nearly half of the total growth in wage and salary jobs between now and 2005. One out of every eight new positions will be education-related. In Projections of Education Statistics to 2007, the National Center for Education Statistics predicts that rising enrollments, combined with increased education revenue from state sources and lower pupil-teacher ratios, will create the need for 350,000 new teaching positions between now and 2007. Former Secretary of Education Richard W. Riley and the National Commission on Teaching and America's Future affirmed that two million jobs will need to be added in the next decade to replace an aging teaching force. The sum of 2.3 million new job openings in the next ten years will be available for today's graduating professionals.

According to Projections of Education Statistics to 2011, public and private elementary and secondary school enrollment peaked in fall 2000 at a record level reflecting an increase of 14 percent since fall 1990. Small enrollment increases are expected between 2000 and 2005, followed by small enrollment declines for most of the years between 2005 and 2011. The continuing increase through 2005 is primarily attributed to the rise in the number of annual births between 1977 and 1990-sometimes referred to as the baby boom echo. Following minor declines and a period of stability from 1991 to 1997, the number of births has begun rising again. Reflecting this, the 3- to 5-year-old population is projected to increase 4 percent by 2011. Increases in the 5- to 13-year-old population from 1999 to 2002 and decreases from 2003 to 2008, followed by slight increases in 2009 to 2011 caused rises in K-8 enrollment in 2001 and expected decreases through 2008 and then increases to 2011. Over the next decade, elementary enrollment is projected to remain at the high levels evident in the late 1990s. Growth in the 14- to 17-year-old population to 2007 and decline through 2011 will continue to influence growth in grades 9 through 12 enrollments through 2006. Between 2000 and 2011 enrollment in secondary schools is projected to exceed enrollment in the late 1990s. Sheer numbers of students who will be enrolled in schools almost guarantees opportunities for teaching careers.

Even though there is a teacher shortage, currently this shortage is not as prominent in Physical Education. However the predicted increases in the numbers of students will likely increase job opportunities for Physical Education teachers.

Advantages and Disadvantages of Teaching

Teaching careers are not noted for extremely high salaries; however, most teachers maintain a good lifestyle. Most individuals who choose to teach do so for a more humane reason: the opportunity to positively affect the lives of young people. Teaching is undeniably a satisfying and rewarding career whether it is in elementary school, middle school, secondary school, or college/university. Teaching offers many perks such as job tenure, medical and life insurance benefits, and frequent and extended vacation time. Tenure provides job security. In most PK-12 school systems, tenure is granted after three years of satisfactory teaching service. On the college/university level, tenure is earned after three to seven years of satisfactory teaching, publishing, and other accomplishments specified by the college/university of employment. Medical and life insurance benefits are generally a part of the benefits packet for teachers. The comprehensiveness of the benefits packet depends upon various factors including the size and location of the educational system. Frequent and extended vacation time is a very attractive benefit of teaching. It provides teachers with the opportunity to travel, to earn additional money, to rejuvenate, or to do whatever they will. In addition to the perks, there are some disadvantages to a teaching career, particularly in physical education. Often there is lack of support from administrators, parents, and community; inadequate facilities, equipment and supplies; and large classes and heavy teaching loads. In spite of the disadvantages, teaching is a challenging and fulfilling career.

Education and Practical Experience

The teaching of physical education is one of the primary roles of physical education majors who graduate from physical education departments in colleges and universities across the country. Teaching physical education in both traditional and nontraditional settings can be an interesting and challenging career. Physical education teachers have the opportunity to work with students in each of the domains: psychomotor, cognitive, and affective. They help students develop motor skills, physical fitness, and a healthy lifestyle. In order to teach you must have the appropriate educational background and practical experiences.

To become a teacher in the traditional school setting requires a minimum of a bachelor's degree. You must meet entry-level requirements to enter the profession. Many states require teacher preparation students to pass a standardized examination and achieve a 2.5 or better (on a 4 point scale) cumulative grade point average to gain admission to and maintain retention in the program. There may also be other requirements such as receiving a passing score on reading and writing proficiency exams. A 2.5 or better grade point average must be maintained cumulatively, and in both the content area and the professional studies area to enter the professional internship. An exit examination may also be required for completion of the program. The exit examination may include teaching a demonstration lesson, a portfolio, a written examination, an interview or any variety of related activities. Upon completion of your curriculum and meeting requirements, you will enter the final phase of preparation for entry into the teaching profession: the professional internship. Examples of the types of courses required in general studies, the content area, and in professional studies are listed in Table 3.1.

The physical education curriculum in Table 3.1 is an example of typical course requirements for a basic teacher certification program. Each university may require different courses and a different number of hours for the completion of the program. Read your college/university catalog and check with your academic advisor for requirements specific to your program.

In addition to the satisfactory completion of coursework, employers look for candidates with work experience and who have a good understanding of what is involved in the job situation. The professional internship is required and is one means of attaining some formal experience. It is an opportunity for you to see how it feels to be a real teacher in a real teaching situation. The internship may last anywhere from twelve weeks to one year. Outside of the formal experiences required in the curriculum, there are many other mechanisms for you to gain valuable applicable experiences. Volunteerism is an excellent way to gain experience. There are opportunities to give of your time in schools and after school programs, with community agencies such as the YMCA/YWCA and Boys and Girls Clubs, with special activities such as Special Olympics and Senior Olympics. There are also opportunities for part time and summer jobs that will give you invaluable experiences and great additions to your resume.

Table 3.1 Physical Education Curriculum

General Studies	Content Area	Professional Studies

English Composition
Introduction to Literature
Humanities (e.g. Art
  Appreciation)
History
General Psychology
World Geography
General Biology
Physical Science
Mathematics
Speech
Personal Health
Orientation
	Physical Fitness &Wellness
	Human Anatomy & Physiology
	Introduction to Physical Education
	Physical Activity Courses:
	  swimming, team sports, dance,
	  individual and dual sports,
	  recreational games
	First Aid and CPR
	Adapted Physical Education
	Theory and Techniques of
	  Coaching & Officiating
	Prevention & Care of Athletic
	  Injuries
	Physiology of Exercise
	Kinesiology
	Physical Activities for the Aging
	Administration of Athletic and
	  Physical Education Programs
	Psychology of Sports & Physical
	  Activity
	Motor Learning
	Motor Development
	Professional Preparation in
	  Physical Education
		Foundations of Education
		Psychology of Learning
		Tests, Measurement, and
		  Evaluation in Physical
		  Education
		Instructional Technology for
		  Educators
		Classroom Management
		Methods of Teaching Elementary
		  School Physical Education
		Methods of Teaching
		  Middle/High School Physical
		  Education
		Professional Internship in PK-12
		  in Physical Education

Professional Competencies

Teacher education programs in physical education are designed to prepare professionals who are equipped to demonstrate a significant degree of success in teaching PN-12 physical education. Students who complete the basic certification program are expected to:

- Contribute to the promotion of behavioral changes that will enhance and maintain an optimal level of lifespan health and fitness.

- Demonstrate a broad-based knowledge in the content areas of physical education.

- Demonstrate an understanding of the principles of and factors affecting growth and development.

- Demonstrate competence in guiding the psychomotor, cognitive, and affective learning in mainstream and special populations.

- Understand the relationship of physical education to other disciplines.

- Formulate and follow developmentally appropriate unit and lesson plans.

- Formulate and select developmentally appropriate activities and instructional materials in physical education.

- Communicate effectively and work cooperatively with students, parents, teachers and administrators.

- Develop research skills through the study of present research and the development of research projects.

From these expectations, six distinct competencies have been identified for mastery. Table 3.2 further explains each competency area. The competency areas are:

- Content
- Instructional delivery
- Classroom management

- Planning and organization
- Assessment and evaluation
- Personal and professional responsibility

Table 3.2   Competencies in Physical Education

Competency Area	Statement of Purpose	Degree Competency
1. Content	Demonstrate competency in the field of Physical Education.	Demonstrate knowledge of and skills in subject matter through the ability to demonstrate a broad-base knowledge in the content area including the performance of psychomotor skills, knowledge of pedagogy, human growth and development, and research.
2. Instructional Delivery	Demonstrate competency in the field of Physical Education.	Demonstrate instructional delivery skills through the ability to (1) teach lessons and (2) employ a variety of teaching methods appropriate to specific learning situations.
3. Classroom Management	Demonstrate competency in the field of Physical Education.	Demonstrate classroom management and discipline skills.
4. Planning and Organization	Demonstrate competency in the field of Physical Education.	Demonstrate planning and organization skills through the ability to (1) follow and formulate developmentally appropriate unit plans, (2) select and formulate developmentally appropriate activities and instructional materials, and (3) formulate a program curriculum.
5. Assessment and Evaluation	Demonstrate competency in the field of Physical Education.	Demonstrate pupil assessment and evaluation skills through the ability to (1) assess and evaluate standard tests and construct valid evaluation instruments for written testing and performance rating; (2) assess and evaluate the general health and fitness status of students.
6. Personal and Professional Responsibility	Demonstrate competency in the field of Physical Education.	Demonstrate personal and professional responsibility through the ability to (1) work with other teachers and professionals to coordinate efforts and make joint program decisions and (2) communicate effectively and work cooperatively with students, parents, teachers, and administrators.

Initial Programs in Physical Education Outcomes

The National Association for Sport and Physical Education/National Council for Accreditation of Teacher Education (NASPE/NCATE) guidelines are based on the National Standards for Beginning Physical Education Teachers. The Beginning Teacher Standards provided the profession with benchmarks by which to measure teacher preparation and serve as organizing centers for reflection on specific components of programs. Current educational thought in the field are clearly linked to NASPE NK-12 Physical Education Standards.

Standard 1: Content Knowledge

A physical education teacher understands physical education content, disciplinary concepts, and tools of inquiry related to the development of a physically educated person. This standard represents the discipline specific content and skill knowledge. To meet this standard, institutions will document assessment activities that include motor skills, content knowledge in sub-disciplines, and the application of disciplinary content to teaching.

Standard 2: Growth and Development

A physical education teacher understands how individuals learn and develop and can provide opportunities that support their physical, cognitive, social and emotional development. The focus of this standard is the application of growth and development concepts to specific teaching experiences. Preservice teachers will demonstrate the ability to plan and implement developmentally appropriate learning experiences based on expected development progressions.

Standard 3: Diverse Learners

A physical education teacher understands how individuals differ in their approaches to learning and creates appropriate instruction adapted to these differences. Through this standard, preservice teachers demonstrate their ability to plan and implement learning experiences that are sensitive to diverse learners.

Standard 4: Management and Motivation

A physical education teacher uses an understanding of individual and grou0p motivation and behavior to create a safe learning environment that encourages positive social interaction, active engagement in learning, and self-motivation. This standard is concerned with preservice teachers' use of a variety of strategies to institute behavior change, manage resources, promote mutual respect and self-responsibility, and motivate students.

Standard 5: Communication

A physical education teacher used knowledge of effective verbal, nonverbal and media communication techniques to foster inquiry, collaboration and engagement in physical activity settings. Preservice teachers will demonstrate the use of assorted media and technology for presentation of lessons, demonstrate sensitivity to all learners and model appropriate behavior and illustrate communication strategies for building a community of learners.

Standard 6: Planning and Instruction

A physical education teacher plans and implements a variety of developmentally appropriate instructional strategies to develop physically educated individuals. This standard deals specifically with pedagogical knowledge and application. The core of this standard will be a series of sequential and progressive field experiences that allow preservice teachers to refine, extend and apply their teaching skills.

Standard 7: Learner Assessment

A physical education teacher understands and uses formal and informal assessment strategies to foster physical, cognitive, social and emotional development of learners in physical activity. Preservice teachers will explore the use of various forms of authentic and formal assessment to guide instruction, provide feedback to candidates, and to evaluate their teaching. Included within this exploration will be an analysis of the appropriateness of various assessments.

Standard 8: Reflection

A physical education teacher is a reflective practitioner who evaluates the effects of his/her actions on others (e.g., learners, parents/guardians, and professionals in the learning community) and seeks opportunities to grow professionally. This standard can be met through a series of learning experiences that promote self-reflection on the part of preservice teachers. Problem solving strategies, self-analysis of lessons and evaluation of program designs could be included in this standard. In addition, preservice teachers should demonstrate a commitment to professional service by involvement in local, state, district and national organizations.

Certification and Advanced Degrees

Teacher certification is required in order to teach in the traditional PK-12 school settings. It is mandated that teachers obtain a valid teaching certificate in the state of employment (See Chapter 5 for credentialing organizations). Certification requires the completion of a teacher certification program at a college or university with an accredited teacher education program. Additionally, passing a standardized examination is required. Some states administer a national examination such as The *Praxis Series: Professional Assessments for Beginning Teachers*, while some states administer a state examination such as the *Alabama Perspective Teachers Test*. The examinations assess basic reading, writing, and mathematics skills that all teachers are expected to have mastered. Additional examinations to measure prospective teachers' knowledge of and skills in their major fields of study may be required. Receipt of the actual teaching certificate requires submission of an application through the university certification officer or the State Department of Education. The process may vary by state.

Advanced degrees are required for college/university level teaching and may be required to advance to a higher step on the salary schedule on the PK-12 level. The educational requirements for teaching physical education in nontraditional settings vary by careers. Some do not require a degree; however, some college and certifications are required. Many of the nontraditional careers require advanced degrees such masters or doctoral degrees.

Colleges and universities offer advanced level degrees in physical education and related areas across the country. Masters and doctoral level programs offer a wide variety of areas of concentration ranging from education to biomechanics to sport history to exercise physiology to administration. Your career of interest will determine which concentration you will pursue. If you are a full time graduate student, the average masters' degree program takes about one year to complete and the doctoral program takes about three years to complete. Just as there are a wide variety of career choices requiring masters and doctoral degrees, there are many that require medical degrees. Medical degrees require substantially more time to complete. In addition to undergraduate school, it takes approximately eight years to complete the degree and fulfill residency requirements.

TEACHING CAREERS IN PHYSICAL EDUCATION

PK-12 School Careers
Elementary School (Pre-Kindergarten - 6th grade)
Middle School (6th - 8th grade)
Secondary School (7th - 12th grade)

Specialized PK-12 School Careers
Adapted Physical Educator
Dance Educator

Post-Secondary School Careers
Junior College
Community College

College/University

Specialized Post-Secondary Careers
Pedagogy Professor
Adapted Physical Education Professor
Biomechanics Professor
Motor Learning Professor
Motor Development Professor
Sport Philosophy Professor
Sports Medicine

Physical Activities Instructor
Sport Management Professor
Exercise Physiologist Professor
Sport Psychology Professor
Sport History Professor
Sport Pedagogy Professor

PK-12 School Careers

Traditional teaching careers in physical education occur in both public and private schools on the PK-12 level. PK-12 School physical education programs are designed to assist students in becoming a "physically educated person." A physically educated person is defined by the National Association for Sport and Physical Education (NASPE) as one who has learned skills necessary to perform a variety of physical activities, is physically fit, participates regularly in physical activity, and knows the implications of and benefits from involvement in physical activity, and values physical activity and its contribution to a healthful lifestyle. PK-12 school physical education careers include:

- Elementary School Physical Educator   • Junior High School Physical Educator
- Middle School Physical Educator   • High School Physical Educator

Elementary School Physical Educator
Elementary school physical educators focus on helping students attain competency in motor skills. Skill development progresses from the introduction of fundamental motor skills and concepts in the early elementary grades to the refinement and combined use of the skills to participate in a variety of developmentally appropriate health-enhancing fitness activities in the upper elementary grades. Elementary school physical educators may teach eight to ten 30-minute classes per day. A Bachelor's degree in physical education and teacher certification are required. The Master's degree is preferred. Salaries for elementary school teachers are based on the salary structure for all teachers in the employing system.

Middle/Junior High School Physical Educator
The middle/junior high school physical educator is responsible for providing systematic instruction in a wide variety of activities that include conditioning and physical fitness, individual and dual sports, team sports, gymnastics, rhythms and dance, track and field, aquatics, outdoor activities. Middle school physical educators teach five to six 50-minute classes per day. They may be required to coach sports teams. A Bachelor's degree in physical education and teacher certification are required. The Master's degree is preferred. Salaries for middle/junior high school teachers are based on the salary structure for all teachers in the employing system. A supplemental salary is provided for coaching duties.

High School Physical Educator
The high school physical educator provides opportunities for students to use a variety of health-enhancing physical activities to reinforce and apply fitness components and concepts. The high school physical educator should reinforce what was learned in earlier grades and teach students how to develop a personal lifelong plan for physical activity. High school physical educators may teach three to five 50 to 90 minute classes per day. They may be required to coach sports teams. A Bachelor's degree in physical education and teacher certification are required. The Master's degree is preferred. Salaries for high school teachers are based on the salary structure for all teachers in the employing system. A supplement salary is provided for coaching duties.

Specialized PK-12 School Careers

Specialized PK-12 teachers require special training in the area in which they teach. These specialists may teach on any level PK-12.

- Adapted Physical Educator   • Dance Educator

Adapted Physical Educator
The adapted physical educator (APE) assists with meeting the physical activity needs of chronically or temporarily disabled students. The APE may be employed at one school or as an itinerant teacher traveling between schools. This specialist may have self-contained adapted classes in which individualized instruction for special needs students are provided or may assist physical education teachers or classroom teachers in meeting the needs of disable students who have been placed in regular classes through inclusion. The APE may be employed on any level PK-12. Salaries for adapted physical educators are based on the salary structure for all teachers in the employing school system. However, itinerant teachers receive a supplement for mileage.

Dance Educator

The dance educator conducts the dance program in schools and is responsible for teaching dance as a performing art. The dance educator should teach a variety of dance forms and include aesthetics, history, and critical analysis of dance. Students should be provided opportunities for aesthetic expression though performance in class and on stage. The dance educator may be employed on any level PK-12. The dance specialist may teach all dance classes in a performance magnet school or the physical educator with interest in dance may teach one or more dance classes per day in the traditional school setting. Salaries for dance educators are based on the salary structure for all teachers in the employing school system.

Post-Secondary School Careers

Post secondary teaching positions may be found in 2-year community and junior colleges and in 4-year colleges and universities. Faculty members may teach activity courses in the service program in which non-majors elect to participate and/or in the majors program that includes courses required by physical education majors. In addition to teaching responsibilities, faculty are required to conduct research, publish articles and books, serve on departmental and college/university committees, advise students, perform community service, consult with state and other organizations, serve in leadership roles in professional organizations. Work hours are somewhat flexible; however, committee meetings, presentations, and other service extend work hours beyond the regular 40-hour week. The master's degree is the minimum degree required to teach on this level. The doctoral degree is preferred and is required for teaching upper level majors' courses in 4-year colleges/universities. Salaries are based on the salary structure of the particular college/university.

Non-School Settings

Examples of teaching in non-school settings include teaching in golf and tennis centers; community recreation programs; Y.M.C.A/Y.W.C.A; and commercial sport clubs such as swim, racquet ball, or gymnastic clubs. The teacher generally works with highly motivated individuals since the participants are voluntary. Many non-school settings require the teacher to teach a diverse number of activities, and there is a lack of job security. Salaries vary widely and working hours may be in the late afternoon or evening and often on weekends. These jobs may be seasonal depending on the nature of the activity and geographic location for teaching of activities such as golf, tennis, and swimming programs.

NON-TEACHING CAREERS IN PHYSICAL EDUCATION

Fitness/Health Careers

Personal Fitness Trainer   Strength Trainer
Health/Fitness Club Manager/Instructor   Corporate Fitness Center Manager/Instructor
Fitness Trainer/Aerobics Instructor   Somatics Instructor
Athletic Clubs/Center Director/Instructor   Weight Management Consultant
Stress Management Consultant

Recreation Careers

Private Clubs Fitness/Activities Instructor   Activities Instructor
Aquatics Specialist   Facility Manager
Commercial Recreation Instructor   Resort Activities Instructor
Camp Instructor or Park Ranger   Sports Club Instructor
Veterans Hospital Recreation Director   Dance Studio Director/Instructor
YMCA/YWCA Activities Instructor   Intramural/Recreational Sports Director
Correctional Facilities Recreation Director   Wilderness Therapy Program Director
Sports Tour Operator   Child-Care Center Instructor
Outdoor Education Instructor   Camp Activities Director/Instructor
Geriatric Fitness Instructor   Church Recreation Instructor
Retirement Center Recreation Director/Instructor   YMCA/YWCA Fitness Instructor

Therapy-Related Careers

Recreational Therapist

Movement Therapist

Physical Therapist

Dance Therapist

Other Related Careers

Professional Dancer

Emergency Services Personnel Instructor

Military Physical Education Specialist

Protective Services Personnel Instructor

Professional Associations/Organizations

Executive Director

Director of Communications

Membership Coordinator

Administrative Assistant

Associate Executive Director

Assistant Director of Administration

Meeting and Event Coordinator

Fitness/Health Careers

The fitness industry has steadily grown over the last two decades, with fitness trainers and aerobics instructors listed as number twenty of the top twenty-five careers projected to grow the fastest from 2000 to 2010. Individuals are more conscious about staying healthy, living longer, and having a better quality of life. If your interest is in assisting others in establishing, realizing, and maintaining their fitness interests, then a career as a fitness professional may be right for you. The fitness profession encompasses a variety of positions. The following are descriptions of a sampling of fitness careers.

- Marketing Director
- Member Services Representative
- Corporate Fitness Center Manager
- Health/Fitness Club Manager
- Exercise Physiologist
- Personal Fitness Trainer
- Nutritionist

Marketing Director

The marketing director is responsible for creating and developing activities that increase membership and sponsorship sales. Depending on the goals of the organization, the social market director will plan, market and direct various events and/or fund-raising activities as dictated by the goals of the organization. A Bachelor's degree in physical education and some management, sales or marketing experience, and knowledge of fund-raising are helpful. Salaries range from $15,000 for part-time positions to the top $30,000, with an average of $22,000.

Member Services Representative

The member service representative is primarily responsible for increasing club membership. The responsibilities include planning membership activities, writing or revising membership policies and regulations, or even working the reception desk. A college degree is not required; however, knowledge of fitness industry is a must. Some knowledge of business or sales is helpful. Salaries range from $15,000 to top $30,000, with an average of $22,000.

Corporate Fitness Center Manager

More and more corporations are providing fitness centers as a benefit to their employees. These fitness centers can be as large as a full fitness club and they need someone to manage them. The corporate fitness center manager oversees the day-to-day operation of the center, hiring and training of employees, and development of fitness programs for company employees. A Bachelor's degree in physical education, sports or recreation and experience in club management are the minimum requirements. Managers may also need some form of national or state fitness certification. Salaries range from $36,000 to $42,000. With a Masters degree the average salary is $50,000- $54,000.

Health/Fitness Club Manager

The health/fitness club manager oversees the day-to-day operation of the health club or gym, coordinates the efforts of all employees, and interacts with the club members and potential members. Unlike the corporate center manager, the club manager's job is tied to the success or failure of keeping an influx of new members. A Bachelor's degree in business or physical education or recreation and experience in management or work in various segments of the health club/fitness industry is an advantage. Any business or financial management experience will be a plus. Salaries range from $20,000 to $60,000, with an average of $40,000.

Exercise Physiologist

The exercise physiologist is concerned with the effects of exercise on the systems of the human body. They study and recommend training methods to help individuals return from injury, improve performance and stay healthy. Their responsibilities are to help individuals determine the proper conditioning programs, the correct methods for developing strength, which exercises are of particular benefit. The Master's or PhD degree in exercise physiology is required. Beyond the advanced degrees and job experience, state licensing and/or board certification is required. Salaries range from $25,000 to $75,000, with an average of $50,000.

Personal Fitness Trainer

The primary function of the personal trainer is to instruct individual clients on the proper methods of exercising according their age and fitness abilities. More than that, the personal trainer has to be skilled individual who can motivate people to want to meet their fitness goals. Most employers, and many clients, will expect the personal trainer to have Personal Trainer Certification. Some clubs may also require a Bachelor's degree in exercise physiology. Experience with various types of exercise equipment and experience as personal trainer for a corporate center or private club will be helpful. Resume Builders. Generally personal trainers are paid by the hour. Pay ranges from $25 - $200 dollars depending on location and experience.

Nutritionist

The nutritionist works with doctors and/or individuals to develop meal plans that will keep them healthy. Nutritionists can influence how individuals improve their physical health such as disease and weight control by manipulating meal preparation and diet. The Bachelor's degree in dietetics, foods and nutrition service management or a related field is a must. A Master's degree or Ph.D. may be required for additional advancement. Nutritionists are required to have state licensing and board certification. A supervised practical experience or an internship will also be required. Salaries range from $20,000 to $75,000, with an average of $45,000.

Recreation Careers

Recreation is considered to be self-chosen activities the revitalize and refresh the body and spirit. The field is experiencing rapid growth and expansion. The number and types of activities have increased, settings in which services are offered have diversified, and the number and range of populations served have expanded. Recreation provides and opportunity for individuals to learn to use their leisure time constructively and in ways that are personally fulfilling. Examples of recreation careers are:

• Facility Manager	• Activities/Sports Instructor
• Director of Intramural/Recreational Sports	• Camp Instructor/Park Ranger
• Wilderness Therapy Program Director	• Sports Tour Operator

Facility Manager

The facility manager coordinators all activities that occur within a recreational facility. Their primary duties include assisting with the establishment and implementation of policies rules and regulations, scheduling classroom and recreational areas, maintaining a functional operating environment, and hiring and supervising employees. A minimum of a Bachelor's degree in a related field is required. A Master's with experience in recreational facility management and other business experience may be required. Salaries range from $40,000, to an average of $55,000, up to $75,000 or more.

Director of Intramural/Recreational Sports

The director of intramural/recreational sports supervises all of a school or facility's recreational sporting activities. Responsibilities include selecting activities that will be offered, developing policies for competition, selecting officials, overseeing the budget, and other duties such as marketing the program and securing sponsorships. A minimum of a Bachelor's degree in a related field is required. A Master's with experience in working in an intramural recreational setting and some management experience may be required. Salaries range from $25,000 to $55,000 or more with an average of $40,000.

Wilderness Therapy Program Director

Wilderness therapy programs are designed to help troubled or disadvantaged youth. The director of the program is responsible for developing and coordination the operational aspects of the program including selecting and assigning field staff and implementing new programs. A minimum of a Bachelor's degree in recreational therapy or a related field and certifications are required. A Master's degree is preferred. Needed experiences include outdoor skills, counseling, safety and first aid, managing outdoor programs. Testing, and background checks will likely be required. Salaries range from $28,000 to$55,000 with an average of $37,000.

Activities/Sports Instructor

The activities/sports instructor may work in a wide range of environments and often works as a freelance consultant. Generally, a formal education may not be required. However, certification as an instructor may be mandatory. The requirements that an activities instructor must meet are to have expertise in one or more activities and have the ability to teach the activity to others. Verbal skills, organization, an outgoing personality, salesmanship, and some business skills are a must. Salaries vary greatly.

Camp Instructor or Park Ranger

The camp instructor or park ranger works in natural settings such as parks and campgrounds. Their role can vary depending on the environment and may include such activities as conducting daily or long-term guided tours, holding public forums, assisting with wildlife studies, assisting with regular maintenance, or helping with security. A Bachelor's degree in recreation or a related area is required. A Master's degree may be required for more advanced work in some areas. Salaries range from an average of $20,000 to a high of $30,000.

Sports Tour Operator

The sports tour operator provides recreational activities for vacationers. Activities may include anything from hiking to fishing to skydiving to tennis. The sports tour operator provides the client with the equipment and instruction for an exciting and safe experience. The operator must have expertise in the skills and locales covered and act as a tour guide. No formal education is required, however, a broad knowledge of recreational, communication, and business skills are important. A bachelor's degree in recreation could prove useful. Salaries depend on the type and number of tours conducted.

Therapy-Related Careers

This area of specialization encompasses a variety of careers. Specialists from these areas usually have a prior professional degree or degrees and training in relevant to their field of choice. Therapy related careers are in demand and include:

- Recreational Therapist   · Movement Therapist
- Physical Therapist   · Dance Therapist

Recreational Therapist

The recreational therapist employ a comprehensive, holistic approach to preventive and rehabilitation services to deliver treatment, education and recreation services to people with disabilities and other health conditions. Therapists use play and other recreational activities to help individuals achieve goals in physical, mental, social and emotional development. Therapists are employed in a broad range of clinical, residential and community-based health and recreation settings. A Bachelor's degree in recreational therapy is required for entry-level employment. Experience in therapeutic settings such as rehabilitation centers and senior citizen centers are helpful. Salaries range from $35,000 to $50,000, with an average of $40,000.

Physical Therapist

The physical therapist is the person who encourages the individual to fight the pain of an injury and come back stronger, faster and better than before. The physical therapist has to have knowledge about injuries, how to evaluate injuries and how to recommend treatment plans. A degree from an accredited physical therapy program is required. Many organizations require the Masters degree. Salaries range from $30,000 to $80,000+, with an average of $50,000.

Movement Therapist

The movement therapist employs movement with persons of all ages to provide the opportunity for personal expression, as well as to develop movement and perceptual skills. The therapist may also work with individuals with impairments to help them learn movement skills. A Masters' degree in movement, dance, recreational therapy or a related field is required. Additional course work in adapted physical education, psychology, health, and counseling; as well as experience in therapeutic settings will enhance marketability. Salaries range from $20,000 to $40,000, with an average of $30,000.

Dance Therapist

The dance therapist employs dance with persons of all ages to help alleviate physical, emotional, and social problems. The dance therapist encourages individuals to recognize and convey their feelings and ideas that they may not be able to express verbally. Therapists are employed in rehabilitation centers, psychiatric hospitals, geriatric programs, and in programs for persons with disabilities. A Bachelor's degree in a related field and dance therapy certification is required. Experience in dance and psychology are needed. Salaries range from $25,000 to $50,000, with an average of $40,000.

Association/Organization Careers

Associations and organizations represent the governing bodies of career fields. Nearly every field has an official association or organization administering it. Major responsibilities of the associations and organizations are to guide the membership in governance, provide professional development and educational opportunities, and represent membership in political matters. Examples of associations and organizations in physical education and related fields are: the National Dance Association, National Association for Sport and Physical Education, American College of Sports Medicine, National Athletic Trainers' Association, American Council on Exercise, and American Association of Leisure and Recreation. Association and organization careers include:

- Executive Director
- Associate Executive Director
- Assistant Director of Administration
- Administrative Assistant

- Director of Communications
- Business Manager
- Membership Coordinator
- Meeting & Event Manager

Executive Director

The Executive Director is in charge of the association staff, is in direct contact with the organization officers and the governing body, and is a decision-maker on association matters and business. A Bachelor's degree in a related field is required. A Masters' or Doctorate degree may be required. Experience in business and association management is necessary. Knowledge of the field, understanding of the politics, and ability to work with a broad range of individuals in the field are required. Salaries range from $50,000 to $250,000, with an average of $150,000.

Associate Executive Director

The Associate Executive Director oversees the day-to-day operation of office personnel, assists with business of the association, serves as the senior administrator for all groups and associations, acts as liaison to board of directors/committee, and is an advisor on convention speakers, activities and sites. A Bachelor or Masters' degree in a related field is required and experience in business and association management is necessary. Salaries range from $50,000 to $125,000, with an average of $85,000.

Assistant Director of Administration

The Assistant Director of Administration plans meetings for major association and affiliate organizations, works with affiliate associations, is the staff liaison to officers, board of directors/executive, and performs miscellaneous office duties relations to staff organization and administration. A Bachelor's degree in a related field and a Masters' degree in a related area or in business administration, communication and computer skills are needed. Salaries range from $35,000 to $65,000, with an average of $50,000.

Administrative Assistant

The Administrative Assistant is responsible for a variety of duties, which include staff liaison to affiliate associations, administering listservs for various associations, daily interaction and supervision of interns, and miscellaneous responsibilities related to office and equipment. A Bachelor's degree in a related field is required, a Master' is desired. Knowledge of the field and prior association experience is required. Salaries range from $25,000 to $40,000, with an average of $30,000.

Director of Communications

The Director of Communications is the primary media contact for the organization, coordination of the web site and all other forms of communication. This job consists of writing, editing, coordinating the editorial calendar, publishing the association magazine, supervising all outgoing materials, preparing speaker scripts and introductions for conventions, and preparing association advertisements. A bachelors' degree in a related field is a minimum requirement. A Master's degree in sports or athletics administration is strongly recommended. Experience as a college/university sports information director or conference information director is helpful. Excellent written, verbal, and computer skill are essential. Salaries range from $50,000 to $100,000 plus, with an average of $75,000.

Business Manager

The Business Manager handles all accounts, employee benefits and payments; processes dues and payments for association and affiliate association memberships; handles staff travel accommodations and oversees registration for conventions, workshops and other events. A degree in business, computer skills and knowledge of accounting software packages is required. Experience as an assistant business manager is helpful. Salaries range from $30,000 to $60,000 plus, with an average of $45,000.

Membership Coordinator

The Membership Coordinator is in charge of all invoices for membership dues, tracks turnover of members and moves, provides membership information to association staff, and updates committee lists and changes in positions. A degree is not required; however, three to five years of experience as membership coordinator may be required. Salaries range from $30,000 to $55,000, with an average of $40,000.

Meeting and Event Manager

The Meeting and Exhibits Manager is responsible for selling exhibits at conventions and workshops, arranging hotel accommodations and transportation for personnel, menus for convention activities, and other miscellaneous items. No degree is required, but experience in the hotel industry, business, and/or catering is needed. Salaries range from $35,000 to $50,000, with an average of $45,000.

THE FUTURE OF PHYSICAL EDUCATION

Making an exact prediction about the future of physical education is not possible, however, as professionals we must undertake preparation to assure that we are not overtaken by future events. One way to plan for the future is to accept the premise of David Bell. Bell points out that time is not an "overarching leap" from the present to the future, but it has its origins in the past, incorporates the present, and extends into the future. In order to make any predictions of the future of physical education, it is necessary for professionals to have knowledge of the past and present as well as understand what the experts are predicting for the future.

In planning for the future, we must recognize that change is ever present and that it occurs at a rapid pace. Certain trends and developments help generate a better understand of the future and the future of physical education. The trends described earlier in this chapter, as well as other developments, are likely to continue to have significant implications for the future of physical education. Wuest and Bucher suggest that as physical educators prepare for the future, they must do the following:

- Provide themselves with the proper credentials to establish jurisdiction over their domain.

- Utilize technological advances to improve the delivery system.

- Prepare for space and underwater living and for changes in our society.

- Become a positive role model for a fit and healthy lifestyle, so that others will be favorably influenced to emulate the lifestyle.

- Help persons to become increasingly responsible for their own health and fitness.

- Recognize that individuals will live longer and become more fit and active in the years to come.

- Provide for all persons, regardless of age, skill, disabling condition, and socioeconomic background, throughout their lifespan.

- Remember that we are all involved with the development of the whole person as a thinking, feeling, moving human being.

- Make a commitment to conduct high-quality programs that are sensitive to individual needs so that physical education's potential to enhance health and quality of life for all people can be achieved.

As the field of physical education continues to expand, the number and types of careers will continue to expand. Physical education professionals must be prepared to create and implement innovative and quality school and non-school programs for an increasingly diverse population in increasingly diverse settings. The future of physical education is coming; it is up to physical educators where it is going.

SUMMARY

Physical education is a comprehensive field that engages individuals of all ages, abilities, and cultures in movement experiences that contribute to their growth and development. Physical education is a dynamic field, constantly evolving as societal trends, demographics, and other factors impact upon it.
The field of physical education offers numerous career opportunities for the professional physical educator. Teaching careers are available both in schools as well as in a wide variety of settings outside of schools. Many related careers in physical education are available. Some of the related careers are in the areas of fitness, recreation, therapy, and with physical education related associations and organizations. As new trends and developments occur and the field continues to expand, more and more career opportunities will present themselves.

REFLECTIONS

1. Using the research data from laboratory 3.1, determine the advantages and disadvantages of a select physical education career and explain why you would or would not choose that particular career.

2. Using the Internet, research three diverse careers in physical education. Decide on two locations where you would like to live and gather details about the availability and salaries in those locations. Use Laboratory 3.2 for your response.

WEB SITES

www.aahperd.org
American Alliance for Health, Physical Education, Recreation and Dance

www.aahperd.org/aalr
American Association for Leisure and Recreation

www.acefitness.org
American Council on Exercise

www.apta.org
American Physical Therapy Association

www.aahperd.org/naspe
National Association for Sport and Physical Education

www.nata.org
National Athletic Training Association

www.nirsa.org
National Intramural and Recreational Sports Association

www.pecentral.org
PE Central

www.joyjobs.com
Teaching Jobs Overseas

www.k12jobs.com
Current k-12 teaching positions

BIBLIOGRAPHY

Allen, B.J. and Floyd, Patricia A. (2007). *Elementary School Physical Education – A Healthful Living Approach*, 2nd ed. Pearson Education.

Brown, M. (1997). Globalize Yourself. *Next Step*. 2:2, 50-52.

Buck, Marilyn; Jable, Tom; Floyd, Patricia A. (2004). *Introduction to Physical Education and Sport: Foundations and Trends*. Belmont, CA: Thomson, Wadsworth.

Lumpkin, A. (2007). *Introduction to Physical Education, Exercise Science, and Sport Studies*, 7th ed. Boston, MA: McGraw-Hill.

NASPE (2004). *Physical Activity for Children: A Statement of Guidelines for Children Ages 5-12*, 2nd ed. Reston, VA: NASPE Publications.

NASPE (2004). *Standards for Initial Programs in Physical Education Teacher Education*. Reston, VA: NASPE Publications.

Siedentop, Daryl (2007). *Introduction to Physical Education, Fitness, and Sport*, 6th ed. Boston, MA: McGraw-Hill.

Wuest, D.A. and Bucher, C.A. (2006). *Foundations of Physical Education and Sport*, 13th ed. Boston, MA: McGraw-Hill.

www.yarrabah.sch.vic.edu.au

LABORATORY ACTIVITY 3.1

NAME _____ DATE _____

COURSE _____ SECTION _____

Interview three persons in three diverse careers in physical education (i.e. secondary school teacher, fitness center aerobics instructor, senior citizen exercise program) to determine their opinion of the advantages and disadvantages of the career. Record your findings below.

LABORATORY ACTIVITY 3.2

NAME _____ DATE _____

COURSE _____ SECTION _____

Using the Internet, research three diverse careers in physical education. Decide on two locations where you would like to live and gather details about the availability and salaries in those locations. Use Laboratory 3.2 for your response.

CHAPTER 4

INTRODUCTION TO CAREERS IN SPORT

"It's not your aptitude, it's you attitude that determines your altitude".
Anonymous

KEY CONCEPTS

1. Physical activities must take place under specific conditions to be classified as sport.
2. Sport has experienced phenomenal growth over the last four decades.
3. High school and college sport represent an enormous part of the sport industry.
4. There are many diverse careers in sport.
5. The diverse careers in sport require a variety of educational and practical experiences.

INTRODUCTION

Sport occupies a huge spot in the hearts of Americans and it has reached prominent icon status in our culture. Millions of Americans participate in sport activities every day as active participants or as spectators. The scope of sport is tremendous. It cuts across every ethnic group, every age group, and every ability group. It incorporates a wide range of recreational, interscholastic, intercollegiate, and professional activities. Sport has become an economic giant. Billions of dollars are spent on facilities, equipment, supplies, and salaries. Sport is "big business." A myriad of career opportunities are available and it takes all kinds of professionals with all kinds of backgrounds to make it work.

Figure 4.1 Sport Careers

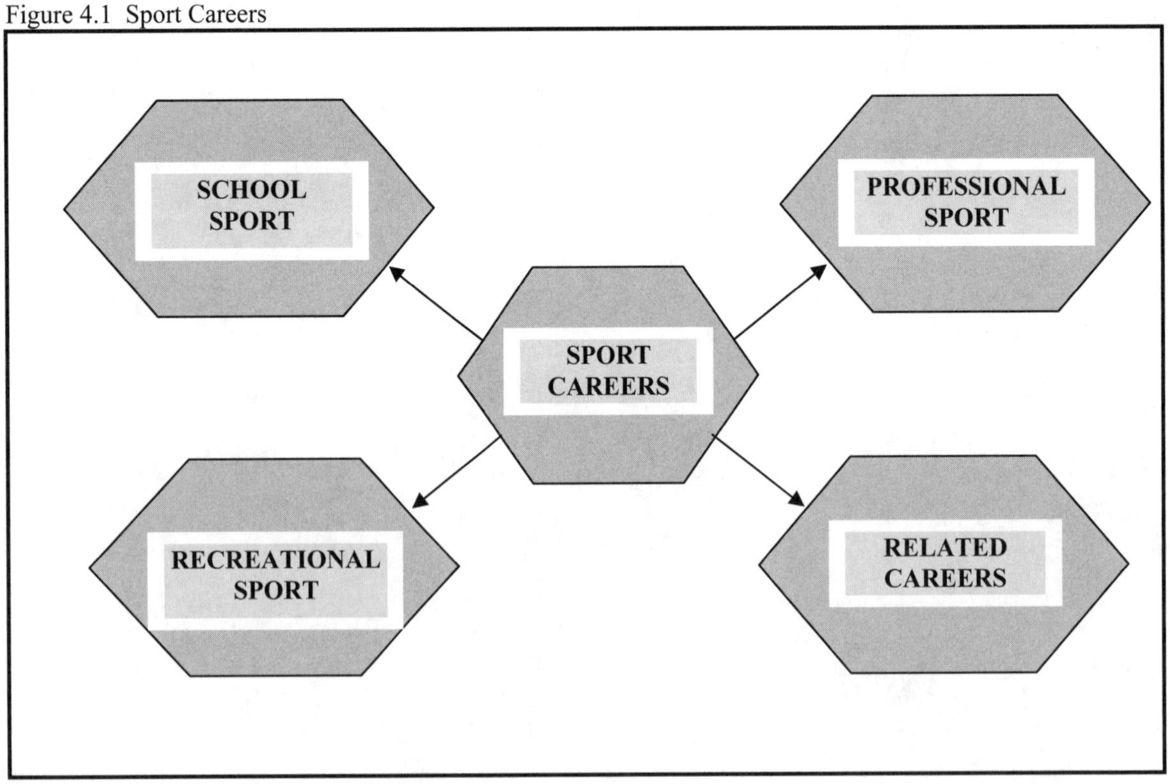

What Is Sport?

Lumpkin broadly defines sport as physical activities governed by formal or informal rules that involve competition against an opponent or oneself and are engaged in for fun, recreation, or reward. Coakley more specifically defines sport as physical activities: that involve vigorous physical skills that require physical exertion, that are institutionalized and competitive, and that involve participants whose participation is both intrinsically and extrinsically motivated. All physical activities that require physical skills and physical exertion cannot be classified as sport. The conditions under which the activity takes place must be considered. Sport sociologists suggest that the physical activity must be competitive, conducted under formal and organized conditions, and must be institutionalized. Competitive physical activity becomes sport when there is standardization and enforcement of the rules governing the activity, there is emphasis on organization and the technical aspects of the activity, and there is a formalized approach to the development skills required to participate in the activity.

Sport is organized, competitive activities that are governed by rules and is meaningful to the participant. People are motivated to engage in sport for many reasons. Some of the reasons are intrinsic and others are extrinsic, they including enjoyment, entertainment, personal satisfaction, and personal reward. Clearly, sport holds many meanings for those who participate and significantly impacts society. Wilkerson asserts that sport has seven functions in society:

- Emotional release – a way to release express emotions, and relieve tension and aggressive tendencies

- Affirmation of identity – opportunity to be recognized and to express individual qualities

- Social control – means of control over people in a society where defiance is prevalent

- Socialization – means of socializing individuals who identify with it

- Change agent – results in social change, new behavior patterns, and changes in the course of history

- Collective conscious – Creates a communal spirit that brings people together for common goals

- Success – provides a felling of success for participants and spectators

CAREER OPPORTUNITIES IN SPORT

Sport has experienced phenomenal growth on every level over the last forty years. We have seen a marked increase in participation in sport by children and youth, the aging, and individuals with disabilities. It is estimated that more than 25 million children and youth participate in organized sport activities outside the school setting through public and private organizations/agencies such as Boys and Girls Clubs and other community organizations, as well as through commercial sports organizations such as gymnasiums and sports clubs. In addition to those participating through community organizations/agencies, there are an increasing number of individuals who elect to participate through amateur sports such as the Amateur Athletic Junior/USA Junior Olympics and US Olympic Festival. There has also been an increase in the number of aging citizens who participate in amateur sports through activities such as the Nation Senior Games/ Senior Olympics and master's competitions. Thousands of senior citizens participate in local, state and national competitions every two years. There are over 50 member organizations with more than 250,000 participants.

In the last two decades, sport opportunities for individuals with disabilities have emerged. The Special Olympics provides opportunities for individuals who are mentally impaired and are eight years of age and older to participate in a variety of sports and games on a local, state, regional, national, and international level. The international organization provides year round training and competition in 26 Olympic-type sports, serves more than 1 million persons in more than 200 programs in more than 150 countries. The number participants are expected to double by year 2005. The Paralympics, recognized by the International Olympic Committee, provides international competition for elite athletes with disabilities. The 2004 Paralympics took place in Athens, Greece following the 2004 Olympics. 4,000 Paralympics athletes from 130 countries, 200 team officials, 3,000 media representatives, 1,000 technical officials, and 15,000 volunteers were to be in attendance.

Participation in sport has also experienced tremendous growth on the interscholastic and intercollegiate levels. Though there continues to be some objections by some educators, sport continues to grow in schools and colleges/universities. According to a recent National Collegiate Athletic Association (NCAA) Participation Study, 3,921,069 youth participate in high school sports and 359,782 college/university students participated in college sports. The growth trend is also reflected in the increase in the number and types of new professional teams.

School Sport Careers

High School Sport Careers

Athletic Director   Assistant Coach
Head Coach   Athletic Trainer

College Sport Careers

Athletic Director   Assistant/Associate Athletic Director
Senior Women's Administrator   Conference Administration
College Coach   Strength & Conditioning Coach
Academic Counselor   Compliance Coordinator
Sports Information Director   Athletic Trainer
Recruiting Coordinator   Equipment Manager
Facilities Manager   Booster Club Coordinator
Marketing Director   Tickets Director
Video Services Coordinator

Professional Sport Careers

Professional Teams

Head Coach   Assistant Coach
General Manager   Facilities Director
Public Relations Director   Director of Corporate Sales
Ticket Operations Director   Community Relations Director
Marketing Director   Promotions Manager
Equipment Manager

Association & Organization Careers

Executive Director   Business Manager
Associate Executive Director   Membership Coordinator
Assistant Director of Administration   Administrative Assistant
Meeting & Event Manager   Receptionist
Director of Communications

Broadcasting & Media Sport Careers

Sports Editor   Sports Writer
Freelance Writer   Graphic Designer
Advertising Sales   Producer
Sports Talk Show Host   Photographer
Affiliate Relations Director   Web Developer

Sports Events Careers

Executive Director   Sales Coordinator
Booking Coordinator   Marketing Manager
Manager of Service Events   Event Coordinator
Public Relations Manager   Staffing Coordinator
Production Engineer   Event Operations

Sporting Goods Careers

Vendor Correspondent

Accountant

Employee Relations Director

Merchandising Analyst

Account Representative

Vendor

Account Executive

Creative Director

Product Manager

Staff Attorney

Marketing Manager

Professional Services Sport Careers

Sports Agent/Athlete Representation

Marketing/Account Management

Risk-Management Insurance

Marketing/Creative

High School Sport Careers

High school athletics represent a large portion of the sport industry. There are more than 17,000 high schools in the United States with athletic programs. The national service administrative organization for high school athletics is the National Federation of State High School Associations. Each state has a state high school athletics association. Today there are over 2.7 million female and more than 2.9 male athletes in America's high schools.

- Athletic Director
- Head Coach
- Assistant Coach
- Athletic Trainer

High School Athletic Director

The High School Athletic Director is responsible for developing the athletic program within the school. The athletic director is responsible for ensuring compliance of athletic rules and regulations, monitoring student eligibility, evaluating programs and coaches, managing program budgets, assisting with the selection of coaching staffs, and attending athletic events. The athletic director may also supervise junior high school coaches whose program feeds the high school. A bachelor's degree in education and a valid teaching certificate are general requirements. The master's degree is preferred. Three or more years of experience as a coach, preferably head coaching, is preferred. Knowledge of budgeting and good organization, management and leadership skills are desirable. A supplemental salary is paid for the position. The supplement is dependent upon the school system in which you are employed.

High School Head Coach

A high school head coach usually becomes a head coach after being an assistant coach at a successful high school program. Responsibilities include overseeing all phases of the program including coaching, monitoring student academics, coordinating team travel, managing program budgeting, promoting the program, hiring and supervising assistant coaches. The head coach is also responsible for assuring that the coaching staff complies with athletic rules and regulations. A bachelors' degree in education is mandatory. Head coaches are required to teach classes; therefore, valid teacher certification is required. Some districts require a Masters degree after given number of years in the school district. Coaching experience on the high school or college level is almost always a must. Volunteer coaching for community and organizations can be helpful. Coaches are paid as teachers. A supplemental salary is paid for coaching. The supplement is dependent upon the school system in which you are employed.

High School Assistant Coach

A high school assistant coach's duties include assisting the head coach in coaching the team, monitoring student eligibility, coordinating team travel, and promoting the program. Assistant coaches may be teachers in the system or volunteers. Requirements are the same as those for a head coach if the assistant coach is a teacher in the system. Volunteer coaches are not required to have a degree or teacher certification. Coaches are paid as teachers. A supplemental salary is paid for coaching. The supplement is dependent upon the school system in which you are employed.

High School Athletic Trainer

A high school athletic trainer's responsibilities include coordinating and carrying out the treatment and rehabilitation of injured athletes and communicating the results to the head coach. Further duties include coordinating physicals for athletes, maintaining medical records for athletes, managing the day-to-day operations of the training room, supervising student trainers, and maintaining and evaluating the equipment to be used by the athletes. A bachelor's degree in education, athletic training, or physical therapy is required, with most schools requiring valid athletic trainer certification from the National Athletic Trainers Association (NATA). Volunteer work as an athletic trainer is helpful. Salaries depend on the school system and the employment level.

College Sport Careers

College sport represents an enormous part of the sport industry. There are over 3,000 colleges and universities in America and nearly all of them have an athletics department. Athletics departments have numerous departments to address the many facets of athletics. The college/university provides opportunities to gain intimate knowledge of sport and an understanding of sport business.

- Athletic Director
- Senior Women's Administrator
- College Coach
- Academic Counselor
- Sports Information Director
- Recruiting Coordinator
- Facilities Manager
- Marketing Director
- Video Services Coordinator

- Assistant/Associate Athletic Director
- Conference Administration
- Strength & Conditioning Coach
- Compliance Coordinator
- Athletic Trainer
- Equipment Manager
- Booster Club Coordinator
- Tickets Director

Athletic Director
The Athletic Director (AD) is the highest executive in the athletic department. The AD is responsible for managing the athletic budget, hiring and supervising coaches and other personnel, scheduling competitions, overseeing facilities, and working closely with alumni. Responsibilities of this position are very similar from the small college to the very large university. A master's degree is required and preference is often given to candidates who hold the doctoral degree. Experience in college athletic administration as an assistant or associate athletic director; strong management, communication, marketing, and finance skills and knowledge of NCAA rules are a necessity. Salaries range from $45,000 to $200,000 plus with an average of $70,000.

Assistant/Associate Athletic Director
The assistant/associate athletic director is the link between the AD and the coaching and department coordinators. The assistant/associate AD works with the department on issues such as staff motivation, budgets and compliance with governing rules and regulations. In addition, keeping the AD informed and aware of the condition of each department is a duty. Some major universities have a several assistant and associate athletic directors while smaller colleges may have one or none. A degree is required and the doctoral degree is preferred. Experience in administration of college athletics is required. Salaries range from $40,000 to $75,000 with an average of $45,000.

Senior Women's Administrator
One of newest positions in college athletics is that of Senior Women's Administrator. The growth of women's sports has created the need for women administrators. The senior women's administrator may serve under the Ad in a capacity similar to the assistant/associate AD or in a position parallel to the AD in the women's athletic program. This position is seen as one of the most significant administrative careers in sports for women. A college degree with a master's or Ph.D. is preferred. The same experiences required by the AD are needed. Salaries range from $45,000 to $200,000 with an average of $75,000.

Conference Administration
Most athletic programs function within a conference structure. A complete staff that services the member institutions runs the conference office. The staff consists of the Commissioner, assistant commissioners, administrative assistant and a variety of other personnel. The conference supervises the overall operations of the conference activities. It is responsible for public relations, broadcasting of games, rules enforcement and compliance, assigning officials, marketing and championships administration. A master's degree is required for the position of Commissioner while a doctorate degree is preferred. Experience in business, budgeting, management, sports administration, and NCAA rules are mandatory. Salaries range from $15,000 to $100,000+ with an average of $60,000.

College Coach

Head and assistant coaching positions for males and females are available on college campuses. At many larger institutions coaches may not be required to teach, however, they may be required to do so at smaller institutions. The major responsibility of a coach is to recruit athletes and prepare them for competition. A masters' degree is required to attain a head coaching position. Head coaching positions require experience in college and/or high school coaching and a winning record. Salaries range from $35,000 to $4 million or more. Bonuses, endorsements and other incentives can raise salaries even higher.

Strength and Conditioning Coach

The strength and conditioning position is a relatively new position within athletics. The strength and conditioning coach is in charge of training athletes to perform at peak levels. Knowledge of physiology, biomechanics, kinesiology, and nutrition is essential in this position. A degree in one of the areas listed or a related area is required and a graduate degree is preferred. Experience working with athletes of both genders and in a variety of sports is recommended. Salaries range from $30,000 to $60,000 with an average of $45,000.

Academic Counselor

Academic counselors work closely with the student-athlete with regard to their academic life. Helping with tutors, study sessions, class schedules, and career guidance are some of the duties of the academic counselor. A masters' degree in academic counseling is required. Experience with academic counseling is required. Salaries range from $24,000 to $45,000 with an average of $35,000.

Compliance Coordinator

The compliance coordinator's job is to ensure that the institution is adhering to the rules and regulations set forth by the NCAA, the NAIA, and the conference in which it competes. This individual must have complete knowledge of all the rules and regulations, rule interpretations, and changes to the rules. Communication with all coaches, student-athletes and administrators is key to the success of program compliance. Experience with athletic departments and compliance are good to have. This position can be a full time position or a part-time position. Many institutions pay a faculty member a supplement for this service. Salaries range from 300,000 to $80,000 with an average of $50,000.

Sports Information Director

The sports information director (SID) is responsible for chronicling the athletic achievements by the institutions teams. The SID prepares press releases and press books, produces program books for games, arranges interviews with the media, and keeps and distributes team and individual statistics. On game day, the SID works with the press to make certain that needed information is available and everything is ready for broadcasting and/or transmitting information to the appropriate source. The sports information staff may consist of one individual with volunteer student assistants in smaller institutions to a staff of many in larger institutions. A degree in journalism or communications is required. Excellent writing and communication skills, knowledge of a variety of sports, and the ability to produce under pressure are desired traits. Salaries range from $18,000 to $60,000 with an average of $40,000.

Athletic Trainer

Athletic trainers are concerned with the health of the athletes. Injury prevention is the main focus of the trainer. If, however an athlete is injured, the trainer is responsible for designing treatment programs and overseeing rehabilitation. On a daily basis the trainer wraps ankles and other body parts, attends to minor injuries, gives massages, and performs numerous other duties. A bachelors' degree in athletic training or a related area and national athletic training certification is mandatory. Experience in athletic training, physical therapy, and injury prevention and treatment is required. Salaries range from $20,000 to $60,000 with an average of $45,000.

Recruiting Coordinator

The recruiting coordinator is responsible for finding and bringing athletes that will produce a championship team into the program. The recruiting coordinator will work with the recruiting staff, professors, administrators and coaches to evaluate candidates for eligibility and scholarships. Recruiting takes patience, insight, the ability to recognize and evaluate athletic skills, and the ability to communicate persuasively. Speaking with teenagers, high school coaches and parents takes a tremendous talent. A college degree combined with coaching experience is necessary. Coaching at the high school or college level, experience in evaluating athletic skill, organizational skills and communication skills are prerequisites. Salaries range from $30,000 to $75,000 with an average of $40,000.

Equipment Manager

All purchasing, maintenance and record keeping of equipment used by the athletic program is the responsibility of the equipment manager. With the help of student volunteers, much of this position becomes budget and inventory control. A bachelor's degree may be required. Experience as a high school or college equipment manager and knowledge of sports equipment is a must. Salaries range from $17,000 to $45,000 with an average of $30,000.

Facilities Management

The facilities manager is in charge of athletic facilities. Duties may include maintenance of the venues and scheduling of activities in the venues. Experience high school, college/university, or other athletic facilities is helpful. Many of the facilities managers have some knowledge of engineering or architecture. Understanding the infrastructure helps in the daily and long term maintenance of a facility. Salaries range from $40,000 to $80,000 with an average of $60,000.

Booster Club Coordinator

The booster Club Coordinator will primarily be responsible for the general well being of the alumni. Alumni, through donations, are responsible for a large part of the money that runs the athletic department. So, keeping the alumni happy is key to continuing the flow of donations to the athletic department. This person will also be responsible for making sure that all contact with the players and donations made to the school follow the NCAA governing rules. The ability to raise funds and function as an administrator is important skills. Salaries range from $17,000 to $75,000 with an average of $40,000.

Marketing Director

The marketing director has to come up with creative ways to fill the seats. In general, the marketing director is responsible for advertising the sports teams competing for the institution. Areas of responsibility include working with local and national media, selling school merchandise, selling tickets and handling public relations events. A masters' degree and experience in business, marketing, or sports administration is preferred. Experience with college/university programs or other marketing experience and knowledge of sports will increase chances of employment. Salaries range from $17,000 to $50,000 with an average of $35,000.

Tickets Director

Any athletic department can produce a great product on the field, have the best staff in the country, but what it comes down to at the end is how many fans were in the seats. The Ticket Manager is responsible all the tickets, the revenue and accounting. The ticket manager is responsible for coming up with season ticket packages, corporate packages, and individual group sales incentives. Creative thinking is required in the development of new marketing strategies for ticket sales. A degree in business, accounting, or a related field is needed. Computer skills, management skills, public relations skills experience are also helpful. Salaries range from $20,000 to $40,000 with an average of $30,000.

Video Services Coordinator

The video services coordinator is responsible for filming all games and practices for use by the coaches and the team. A degree is not required; however, experience in the operation of video equipment and editing machines a mandate. Salaries range from $12,000 to $35,000 with an average of $25,000.

Professional Sport Careers

Professional sport teams are the most widely recognized industry segment. A variety of teams, leagues, and governing bodies make up the professional sport industry. The National Football League, National Hockey League, Women's National Basketball Association, and Arena Football are examples of professional leagues.

- Head Coach
- General Manager
- Public Relations Director
- Ticket Operations Director
- Marketing Director
- Equipment Manager

- Assistant Coach
- Facilities Director
- Director of Corporate Sales
- Community Relations Director
- Promotions Manager

Head/Assistant Coach

Head and assistant coaching positions in professional sports are limited. Responsibilities include practice planning, administrative and public relations, budgeting, player relations, and competition management and strategy. The major responsibility of a coach is to recruit athletes and prepare them for competition. A masters' degree is required to attain a head coaching position. Head coaching positions require experience in college and/or high school coaching and a winning record. Salaries range from hundreds of thousands of dollars to $1,000,000 or more. Bonuses, endorsements and other incentives can raise salaries even higher.

General Manager

The General Manager (GM) of a professional sports team directs the day-to-day operations of the individual divisions that make the team function. The GM is responsible for assuring that every department from administrative affairs, to public relations, to promotions, works as a separate entity and that they work together as a whole. A master's degree in sports or business administration or a related field is recommended. Experience in as many levels of a professional sports organization as possible is critical in developing the skills need to be a successful GM. Excellent administrative skills and the ability to work with a wide variety of people are necessary. Salaries range from $50,000 to $250,000 plus with an average of $75,000.

Facilities Director

The Facilities Director makes sure that every aspect of the sport facility is operating properly, from the lights to the field to the concession stands. A master's degree in sports or business administration or other related field is recommended. Excellent organizational skills and prior facility operations experience are required. Salaries range from $30,000 to $150,000 plus with an average of $60,000.

Public Relations Director

The Public Relations Director is responsible for publicizing the organizations' news and activities. Duties include writing press releases, producing publications, and organizing press box activities. Other responsibilities may include developing web-site content and supporting radio and television broadcasting. A bachelor's degree in sports or business administration, public relations or a related field is required. A master's degree is recommended. Experience in public relations, excellent computer and writing, and verbal skills are mandatory. Salaries range from $35,000 to $75,000 with an average of $50,000.

Director of Corporate Sales

The Director of Corporate Sales is responsible for generating revenue from sources other than the fan base. The director develops partnerships with successful businesses. These partnerships include the luxury skyboxes and sponsorship packages that include signage, advertising, promotions and hospitality. The director's game-day tasks may also involve producing public announcement scripts, TV production, execution of promotions, and game entertainment. A master's degree in sports administration is required. Experience in sales and negotiation skills are also helpful. Salaries range from $30,000 to $75,000 with an average of $50,000.

Ticket Operations Director

The Ticket Operations Director oversees all aspects of ticket sales for the organization. Responsibilities include sales of single-game tickets, season ticket packages, sales of loge boxes, club seats and luxury skybox tickets. The tickets staff also handles duplicate ticket and security problems, will-call booths and the transfer of season tickets. A bachelor's degree in sports or business is recommended. Experience in ticket sales, computer applications, and multi-tasking are good to have. Salaries range from $30,000 to $75,000 plus with an average of $45,000.

Community Relations Director

The Community Relations Director represents the organization's interests to those people who don't read the sports page or attend games. Working to ensure that the community sees the team as an asset and not a liability is the job of the community relation's director. The department works to develop bonds with public entities through events such as charity events, festivals, and other community activities. A bachelor's degree in sports or business administration, public relations or a related field is required. A master's degree is preferred. Experience in public relations, writing, and communication skills are helpful. Salaries range from $25,000 to $75,000 with an average of $50,000.

Marketing Director

The Marketing Director is responsible for selling a professional team to the public. The marketing director oversees all aspects of the team's outside sales from advertising to merchandising and produce development. The director must know how to introduce their product, in this case a name and logo, to the public and make the team attractive to buyers. A bachelor's degree in sports or business administration, marketing or a related field is required. A master's degree is preferred. Experience in sports marketing is required. Excellent communication, public relations, and sales skills are necessary. Salaries range from $30,000 to $75,000 with an average of $50,000.

Promotions Manager

The Promotions Manager must help attract fans by building an exciting and fun atmosphere around the game. Though never as important as the game itself, the atmosphere surrounding a professional event can play a vital part in attracting fans. Promotional tasks include creating, planning, coordinating and executing game-day activities. Sales and implementation of promotional activities must be coordinated with other divisions within the organization such as the sales and communications department. A bachelor's degree in sports or business administration, marketing or a related field is required. A master's degree is preferred. Experience in promotions is needed. This position requires innovativeness, good business sense, and organizational skills. Salaries range from $30,000 to $75,000 plus with an average of $50,000.

Equipment Manager

Making a professional team look professional is the job of the Equipment Manager. From headgear to uniforms, the equipment manager must ensure that the team is well stocked and prepared. The equipment manager keeps abreast of the latest technological advancements in gear. The manager also handles all the logistics for transporting the entire inventory to the game site. A bachelor's in sports or a related field is recommended. Experience as an equipment manager is helpful. Knowledge of sports trends and technology is a plus. Salaries range from $20,000 to $50,000 with an average of $30,000.

Association/Organization Careers

Associations and organizations represent the governing bodies of career fields. Nearly every field has an official association or organization administering it. Major responsibilities of the associations and organizations are to guide the membership in governance, provide professional development and educational opportunities, and represent membership in political matters. Examples of associations and organizations in sport are: National Collegiate Athletic Association, National Federation of State High School Associations, National Association for Girls and Women in Sport, Women's Sports Foundation, National Athletic Trainers' Association, and the National Youth Sports Coaches Association.

- Executive Director
- Associate Executive Director
- Assistant Director of Admin.
- Meeting & Event Manager
- Director of Communications

- Business Manager
- Membership Coordinator
- Administrative Assistant
- Receptionist

Executive Director

The Executive Director is in charge of the association staff, is in direct contact with the organization officers and the governing body, and is a decision-maker on association matters and business. A Bachelor's degree in a related field is required. A Masters' or Doctorate degree may be required. Experience in business and association management is necessary. Knowledge of the field, understanding of the politics, and ability to work with a broad range of individuals in the field are required. Salaries range from $50,000 to $250,000, with an average of $150,000.

Associate Executive Director

The Associate Executive Director oversees the day-to-day operation of office personnel, assists with business of the association, serves as the senior administrator for all groups and associations, acts as liaison to board of directors/committee, and is an advisor on convention speakers, activities and sites. A Bachelor's or Masters' degree in a related field is required and experience in business and association management is necessary. Salaries range from $50,000 to $125,000, with an average of $85,000.

Assistant Director of Administration

The Assistant Director of Administration plans meetings for major association and affiliate organizations, works with affiliate associations, is the staff liaison to officers, board of directors/executive, and performs miscellaneous office duties relations to staff organization and administration. A Bachelor's degree in a related field and a Masters' degree in a related area or in business administration, communication and computer skills are needed. Salaries range from $35,000 to $65,000, with an average of $50,000.

Administrative Assistant

The Administrative Assistant is responsible for a variety of duties that include staff liaison to affiliate associations, administering listservs for various associations, daily interaction and supervision of interns, and miscellaneous responsibilities related to office and equipment. A Bachelor's degree in a related field is required, a Master' is desired. Knowledge of the field and prior association experience is required. Salaries range from $25,000 to $40,000, with an average of $30,000.

Director of Communications

The Director of Communications is the primary media contact for the organization, coordination of the web site and all other forms of communication. This job consists of writing, editing, coordinating the editorial calendar, publishing the association magazine, supervising all outgoing materials, preparing speaker scripts and introductions for conventions, and preparing association advertisements. A bachelors' degree in a related field is a minimum requirement. A Master's degree in sports or athletics administration is strongly recommended. Experience as a college/university sports information director or conference information director is helpful. Excellent written, verbal, and computer skill are essential. Salaries range from $50,000 to $100,000 plus, with an average of $75,000.

Business Manager

The Business Manager handles all accounts, employee benefits and payments, processes dues and payments for association and affiliate association memberships, handles staff travel accommodations and oversees registration for conventions, workshops and other events. A degree in business, computer skills and knowledge of accounting software packages is required. Experience as an assistant business manager is helpful. Salaries range from $30,000 to $60,000 plus, with an average of $40,000.

Membership Coordinator

The Membership Coordinator is in charge of all invoices for membership dues, tracks turnover of members and moves, provides membership information to association staff, and updates committee lists and changes in positions. A degree is not required, however, three to five years of experience as membership coordinator may be required. Salaries range from $30,000 to $55,000, with an average of $40,000.

Meeting and Event Manager

The Meeting and Exhibits Manager is responsible for selling exhibits at conventions and workshops, arranging hotel accommodations and transportation for personnel, menus for convention activities, and other miscellaneous items. No degree is required, but experience in hotel industry, business, and/or catering is needed. Salaries range from $35,000 to $50,000, with an average of $45,000.

Broadcasting & Media Sport Careers

Sports media is defined as the news and events surrounding the world of sport. In addition to newspapers, sports media has evolved to include magazines, radio shows, television shows, and Internet sites and other forms. A variety of opportunities are available in a variety of media forms.

- Sports Editor
- Freelance Writer
- Advertising Sales
- Sports Talk Show Host
- Affiliate Relations Director

- Sports Writer
- Graphic Designer
- Producer
- Photographer
- Web Developer

Sports Editor

The sports editor of a newspaper or magazine is responsible for planning the organizations coverage of the events and teams in their area and across the nation. The sports editor must be able to manage deadlines and plan for breaking news, specials and day-to-day coverage. A master's degree in journalism, English or other related field, and excellent writing and communication skills is required. Experience in writing, editorial skills, and field reporting are a prerequisites. Salaries range from $10,000 to $150,000 with an average of $50,000.

Sports Writer

Sports writers cover a broad range of sports events, from high school to college to the professionals. Writers attend and report on games. They act as the eyes and ears of the fans from the start of preseason through the final play of the year. Sports writers bring game details, behind-the-scene reports, and analysis of coaches, players and organizations to the public. A bachelors' degree in journalism, English, or a related field is required. The masters' degree is preferred. Experience with writing for a magazine, newspaper, or television segment is needed. The ability to adhere to deadlines and adapt to a life on the road is mandatory. Salaries range from $10,000 to $100,000 with an average of $35,000.

Freelance Writer

Freelance writers work independently, selling their services to established clients or to the highest bidder. Freelancing is risky, as the freelancer is never guaranteed that work will be available. Many freelancers spend years working within the industry before branching out on their own. When considering this option, numerous contacts with Internet sports sites, magazines and other media should be well established. Also, investigate the requirements needed to open and operate your own business. The minimum educational requirement is a bachelor's degree in journalism, English or other related field. Freelancers need experience in writing for a magazine, newspaper, television segment, etc. Salaries range from $10,000 to $100,000 with an average of $35,000. Salaries vary according to number and type of jobs.

Graphic Designer

Graphic artists use technology to create enticing and exciting graphic images in newspapers, magazines, web sites and other media. It is the job of the graphic artist to use his/her creativity and skill to make pages that fans find appealing and will want to consume. A bachelor's degree in graphic arts and web design are mandatory. Training and experience with software packages is a must. Knowledge of sports is always helpful. Salaries range from average $45,000 to $75,000 plus.

Advertising Sales

Sports related media relies heavily on advertising sales to keep a publication or show in business. A career in sales could provide an avenue in the sports media world. Selling advertisement requires managing current accounts and developing new accounts. Advertisement sales executives must be personable, organized, sensitive to client demands, and creative with seeking out new sources of revenue. Having knowledge of sports helps when looking for new leads and dealing with the sports industry. A minimum of a bachelor's degree in advertising, journalism, English or related field is needed. Prior advertising experience and good communication skills increase marketability. Salaries range from $25,000 to $75,000 with an average of $50,000.

Sports Talk Show Host

The sports talk show host has to have opinions and be able to relate them to the public in an entertaining manner. Hosting a sports show requires long hours of preparation and organization to make a show interesting and lasting. Talk shows can be produced on television, radio, or the Internet. Show may be broadcast locally, regionally or nationally. A bachelor's degree in journalism or other related field, broadcasting, or a related field is required. Good interpersonal communication skills and experience with talk shows is helpful. Salaries range from $25,000 to $150,000 with an average of $75,000.

Producer

The producer of a television or radio show serves as the department's team leader. Keeping stories and programs on schedule, managing the budget, and finding new sources for stories are few of the responsibilities that producers must handle. They also set the department's standards of operations and assure that those standards are followed. Diligent effort, organization, and creativity are required to keep a sports show entertaining and profitable. A bachelor's degree in media arts, journalism or other related field is needed. Experience in television and radio production is required. Salaries range from $25,000 to $250,000 plus with an average of $75,000.

Affiliate Relations Director

An affiliate relations director is responsible for representing the interests of the network to the individual stations that carry their product. Affiliate relations directors seek out new stations that fit the demographic of their programming, work closely with existing stations to assure that network objectives are being met, and assist in the development of new programs that will be attractive to more stations. A business degree and knowledge of technical requirements are an essential. Experience working with advertisers and representing affiliate stations, good communications and interpersonal skills are required. Salaries range from $35,000 to $100,000 plus with an average of $50,000.

Sports Photographer

Sports photographers tell a story with pictures. The photographer's duty is to bring fans closer to a big moment or a prominent place through the eyes of the camera. Many times a photograph better captures a particular sports moment than any other form of media. A degree may not be required, however, knowledge of sports and experience in sports photography are vital. Salaries range from $12,000 to $55,000 plus with an average of $30,000.

Web Developer

Growth of Internet based sports information has created a wide range of alternative opportunities for experienced people in print or other electronic media. Web developer may be seen as similar to the sports editor at a daily paper or the producer of a sports radio show. The developer is responsible for planning and updating sports sites like newspaper satellites or college athletic departments. A bachelor's degree in graphic or web design or other related field is required. Experience in designing web sites is necessary. Salaries range from $40,000 to $100,000 with an average of $60,000.

Sports Events Careers

Thousands of sporting events are held around the world. Millions of dollars are spent on these events and large staffs are required to manage them. An organizing committee or an event management company runs most events. Event management includes planning and implementing the event and involves everything from client services, to promotional campaigns, to marketing, to sales, sponsorships, to audio/video production.

- Executive Director
- Booking Coordinator
- Manager of Service Events
- Public Relations Manager
- Production Engineer

- Sales Coordinator
- Marketing Manager
- Event Coordinator
- Staffing Coordinator
- Event Operations

Executive Director

The Executive Director oversees the full-time staff, provides direction for event selection and operation, and is decision-maker on organization matters and business. A bachelor's or masters' degree in a related field such as business administration is needed. Experience in association management, meeting planning, contract negotiations, and corporate sponsorships are helpful. Professional or intercollegiate sports experience, knowledge of the industry and the ability think creatively is also helpful. Salaries range from $75,000 to $150,000 with an average of $100,000.

Sales Coordinator

The Sales Coordinator sells venue space to the clients. A bachelor's degree in related field and a master's degree in sports or business administration are required. Experience in sales, event management, knowledge of the industry, professional or intercollegiate sports is useful. Salaries range from $25,000 to $45,000 with an average of $30,000.

Booking Coordinator

The Booking Coordinator schedules events, issues contracts, and distributes booking sheets to clients. A bachelors' or masters' degree in sports, business administration or a related field is required. Experience in sales, professional or intercollegiate sports, and knowledge of the different departments are required. Salaries range from $20,000 to $35,000 with an average of $30,000.

Marketing Manager
The Marketing Manager sells space in a venue or seeks out new events for the organization to coordinate, assists with advertising placement, and coordinates advertising and promotions of pre-event effort. A bachelors' degree in marketing or journalism, and master's degree in Sports Administration or Business Administration are required. Experience in event promotion and marketing with event or sports related organizations are needed. Salaries range from $25,000 to $50,000 with an average of $35,000.

Manager of Service Events
The Manager of Service Events oversees the entire range of events that take place in a venue. Numerous events or large multi-faceted events may be scheduled simultaneously. All the event managers are ;under the supervision of the manager of service events. A master's degree in business education, sports management, or a related area is recommended. Experience in management, professional or intercollegiate sports, and extensive knowledge of the industry are critical. Salaries range from $30,000 to $50,000 with an average of $40,000.

Event Coordinator
The Event Coordinator works with clients to organize and manage events, secure and submit contracts, estimate budgetary, equipment and personal needs, and distributes work orders to the departments. A master's degree in business education, sports management, or a related area is recommended. General business knowledge, budget experience, event planning and operations are a requirement. Salaries range from $20,000, to $40,000 with an average of $30,000.

Public Relations Manager
The Public Relations Manager publicizes upcoming events; gauges and responds to issues arising at events, provides information to media during events; and coordinates activities of outside public relations entities during events. A bachelor's degree in public relations or journalism and a master's degree in sports administration or public relations is required. Experience working as a public relations assistant for college or pro teams, event coordination, and community relations are good to have. Salaries range from $25,000 to $40,000 with an average of $35,000.

Staffing Coordinator
The Staffing Coordinator secures volunteer and paid staffing for events; coordinates efforts of security, ushers, and other service positions; and develops a budget for staffing requirements. A masters' degree in business or sports management and a background in a related area are crucial. Experience with event planning, management, and sports are needed. Salaries range from $20,000 to $40,000 with an average of $35,000.

Event Operations Coordinator
The Events Operations Coordinator is responsible for the field crew, which is responsible for setup and breakdown of seating, flooring, room spacing, etc. of the arena, stadium, or field. A bachelor's degree in related field and experience on staff of a large arena or stadium is useful. Salaries range from $18,000 to $25,000 with an average of $20,000.

Sporting Goods Careers

- Vendor Correspondent
- Accountant
- Employee Relations Director
- Merchandising Analyst
- Account Representative
- Vendor

- Account Executive
- Creative Director
- Product Manager
- Staff Attorney
- Marketing Manager

Vendor Correspondent
A Vendor Correspondent works with vendors on accounts payable, reconciles accounts, and verifies overdue balances. A bachelor's degree in business or accounting is required. Experience in accounting and retail sporting goods sales are excellent resume builders. Salaries range from $15,000 to $25,000 with an average of $20,000.

Account Executive
An Account Executive develops and maintains accounts with outside vendors, constructs and implements new promotional campaigns, and coordinates internal product planning. A bachelor's degree in business marketing is mandatory; a master's degree in business administration or sports administration is strongly suggested. Experience in retail sales or manufacturing is helpful. The ability to develop new clients, generate leads, and communicate well are needed skills. Salaries range from $25,000 to $50,000 with an average of $35,000.

Accountant
An Accountant is responsible for managing accounts, coordinating reports to separate divisions, and developing projects. A bachelor's degree in accounting or related field is required. Work with, accounting, management, accounting software sporting goods manufacturing and sports teams are excellent experiences required. The ability to communicate well prepare written reports are mandatory. Salaries range from $40,000 to $70,000 with an average of $45,000.

Creative Director
A Creative Director is responsible for developing graphic representations of company product lines and creating and implementing plans for the introduction of new product lines. A bachelors' degree in graphic arts, marketing or a related field is mandatory. Experience working with manufacturing, creative development, computer design and word processing software are a necessity. Salaries range from $25,000 to $50,000 with an average of $35,000.

Employee Relations Director
The responsibilities of an Employee Relations Director are to select, lead and manage teams of human resource specialists, develop and implement company policies related to workforce management, and conduct training of new employees regarding workforce relationships. A bachelor's degree in business or human relations or a related field is required. Experience human resources, employee relations, and supervision are needed. Salaries range from $35,000 to $40,000 with an average of $40,000.

Merchandising Analyst
The primary job responsibilities of a Merchandising Analyst are to develop and maintain company merchandising, assist in the implementation of automated reporting systems, gather and distribute reports and assist with planning for new programs. A master's degree in finance, accounting or business or a related field is required. Experience with data analysis and merchandising are needed. Salaries range from $30,000 to $40,000 with an average of $35,000.

Marketing Manager
The primary job responsibilities of the Marketing Manager are to evaluate and implement marketing opportunities, maximize current product lines, and manage budget and workforce in increasing sales of product. A bachelor's degree in marketing is a requirement. Experience as a product or project manager in a marketing organization and work experience within the marketing department of sporting goods manufacturer is helpful. Salaries range from $35,000 to $50,000 with an average of $45,000.

Account Representative
The primary job responsibilities of an Account Representative is to maintain and maximize product sales within a specified region, develop new clients within the region, conduct training after sales, and conduct sales at trade shows. A degree in sales, sports administration or business is required. Experience as a territory salesperson, retail sales, and sports are helpful. Salaries range from $20,000 to $40,000 with an average of $35,000.

Staff Attorney
The primary job responsibilities of the Staff Attorney is to provide general and legal counsel in support of company interests, provide consultation in areas of contract and licensing negotiation, and analyze, prepare and research matters for various company needs. A law degree and licensing in state where the company conducts business is compulsory. Experience as staff attorney for a corporation or in a large law firm and contract negotiations is recommended. Salaries range from $65,000 to $85,000 plus with an average of $75,000.

Product Manager
The primary job responsibilities of the Product Manager are to develop effective programs for sales of current a products, work within the budget to maintain or increase product sales levels, communicate sales needs to the territory, and implement new marketing programs to new markets. A bachelor's degree in sales, marketing or a related field is required. Experience as a territory salesperson, representative in a marketing firm or manufacturer's marketing department is recommended. Salaries range from $20,000 to $30,000 with an average of $25,000.

Vendor
The vendor is responsible for retail sales of sporting good products. No degree is required. Experience in retail sales and business management is required.

Professional Services Sport Careers

The rapid and humongous growth of the sports industry has forced professional service organizations to employ more business professionals that are common to all business industries. Many diverse services are necessary to run the industry. Opportunities for sports law specialists, accountants, graphic designers, information system managers, and a host of other are available.

- Sports Agent/Athlete Representation
- Marketing/Account Management
- Risk-Management Insurance
- Marketing/Creative

Sports Agent/Athlete Representation
The main job of the sports agent is contract negotiation. The role is often extended to include financial consulting and endorsement representation. Depending on the type of representation offered, an agency might do everything for athletes from negotiating a contract and arranging promotional appearances to investing income and preparing taxes. While not an absolute must, a law degree is generally required and provides the expertise needed when reviewing and negotiating contracts. Extensive knowledge of the sports industry, excellent communication skills, and a background in business are minimum skills needed for success. Salaries are dependent upon the sport, the athletes you represent, or the agency of employment. Salaries may begin at $50,000 or more for the beginning agent, while more experienced agents earn percentages of their client's multi-million dollar contracts.

Marketing/Account Management
Marketing companies are designed to handle the promotional needs of sports organizations and other companies. Senior account supervisor is the lead position in the marketing firm. The marketing firm implements the company's strategy relative to all of the events, teams, leagues and companies they represent. Marketing organization's functions can be as broad as developing and implementing the promotions for a professional sports team or as narrow as conducting a promotional ticket giveaway for one event. Some services may be geared toward creative development while others may focus on sales. A bachelor's degree in marketing is required while a master's degree in business administration or sports administration is beneficial. Experience in marketing and management, knowledge trends in marketing, sales and the sports industry are required. Salaries range from $18,000 for coordinators, to $60,000 for account supervisors, up to $100,000 plus for senior account supervisors.

Marketing/Creative
The goal of a sports marketing firm is to develop a plan to help its clients improve their image, sell more tickets, attract sponsors, find participants and any number of other things that increase their income. The creative department of the marketing firm comes up with the slogan or logo to implement the promotional plan. The creative department consists of a creative director who is responsible for building a team that consists of conceptors who produce ideas, copywriters who put the ideas into words, and graphic artists who create visual images from the ideas. The process requires a thorough understanding of the organization and its clients. A bachelors' degree in the field of expertise is expected. Experience with management or creative training in marketing, and other appropriate areas are good training. Salaries range from $18,000 to $60,000 for lower level positions, to $100,000 plus for creative directors.

Risk Management/Insurance

Professionals in the risk management insurance industry provide facilities, teams and individuals with coverage in the event of an accident in the sports venue. The account executive works directly with individual athletes, teams and facilities to evaluate the risk and need for insurance. They also write policies to cover the cost of special prize money such as million-dollar hole-in-one events and losses due to weather such as rained out annual golf tournaments. A bachelor's degree in business, special training and licensure may be required. Experience in the insurance industry and in sports could prove useful. Salaries range from $18,000 to $30,000 with an average of $25,000.

THE FUTURE OF SPORT

It is expected that major advancements will occur in the future of sport. Youth sports will continue to expand. It is possible that youth sport could revert to a more play-oriented design. However, with the current corporate dominance in sport, the economic implications, and the media; youth sport will likely follow the more aggressive capitalistic model. High school and collegiate sports will move forward with more opportunities for women and minorities to participate on all levels. More women will become involved on nearly every level of sport from player to owner. Women's sport will generate revenue, therefore; there will be more career opportunities in women's sport. Opportunities for the aging and people with disabilities will also continue to grow.

Globalization will affect sport on many levels. Countries around the world will collaborate and cooperate to produce international sport events. The Olympics and other international competitions will gain greater importance. Professional sport will continue to be corporate-dominated and the number of professional teams will increase worldwide. New and unique sports will evolve and lesser known sports form other countries will gain exposure and take root in the United States and around the world. The future of sport will continue to be impacted by the changing society. Values, politics, and economics are just a few of the change agents that will influence the evolution of sport. Dominant values will maintain their influence, of course with some influence from newly developing values. Competition is an engrained element of the American value system that directly reflects the business world. As long as extrinsic rewards are a part of the incentive, competition will be a part of the value system.

SUMMARY

Sport has experienced phenomenal growth over the past forty years with increases in participation by children and youth, girls and women, the aging, and individuals with disabilities. People will continue to participate in sport for numerous reasons, whether it is as an active participant or as an observer, for entertainment or for personal reward. It is expected that sport will continue to expand and to have a significant impact on society as we move into the future.

Sport offers a myriad of career opportunities for professionals in many areas of academic preparation. It is important to understand that it takes all kinds of professionals to operate the sport industry. Some of the sport related careers include high school and college/university athletics, professional sports, broadcasting and media, sports venues, sporting goods, sports events, professional services, and sport associations and organizations. As sport expands, more career opportunities will become available.

REFLECTIONS

1. Using the research data from laboratory 4.1, determine the advantages and disadvantages of a select sport career and explain why you would or would not choose that particular career.

2. Reflect upon your experiences in sports (athlete, coach, etc.) and the information in this chapter to determine the advantages and disadvantages of a selected sport career and explain why you would or would not choose that particular career.

WEB SITES

www.acsm.org
American College of Sports Medicine

www.aahperd.org/naspe
National Association for Girls and Women in Sports

www.nata.org
National Athletic Trainers Association

www.ncaa.org
National Collegiate Athletic Association

www.nfshsa.org
Nation Federation of State High School Associations

www.onlinesports.com
Online Sports Center

www.allsports.com/careers/
Sports Careers

www.womensportfoundation.org
Women's Sports Foundation

www.sirc.ca/
Sports Information Resource Center

www.womensportsjobs.com
Sports jobs for females

http://fatty.law.cornell.edu/topics/sports.html
Sports Law materials

BIBLIOGRAPHY

Coakley, J. (2001). *Sport in Society: Issues and Controversies.* Boston, MA: McGraw-Hill.

Lumpkin, A. (2007). *Introduction to Physical Education Exercise Science, and Sport Studies*, 7th ed. Boston, MA: McGraw-Hill.

Ryan, R. (1998). The road to career success. *1999 Job Choices, 42nd ed.* 10-12.

Siedentop, Daryl (2007). *Introduction to Physical Education, Fitness, and Sport*, 6th ed. Boston, MA: McGraw-Hill.

Wilkerson, M. (1996). Explaining the presence of men coaches in women's sports: the uncertainty hypothesis. *Journal of Sport & Social Issues. 20(4):411-26.*

Wuest, D.A. and Bucher, C.A. (2006). *Foundations of Physical Education*, 15th ed. Boston, MA: McGraw-Hill.

LABORATORY ACTIVITY 4.1

NAME _____ DATE _____

COURSE _____ SECTION _____

Interview three persons in three diverse careers in sport to determine their opinion of the advantages and disadvantages of the career. Record your findings below. Use Laboratory 4.1 to record your findings.

LABORATORY ACTIVITY 4.2

NAME _____ DATE _____

COURSE _____ SECTION _____

Arrange with the venue manager to visit a local sport venue on game day. Observe the preparation for the game, activities during the game, and close out after the game. Use Laboratory 4.2 to write up what you observed.

LABORATORY ACTIVITY 4.3

NAME _____ DATE _____

COURSE _____ SECTION _____

Contact a professional sport team and request job descriptions for two or three positions within their organization. Review the descriptions and discuss them with the class. Use Laboratory 4.3 or your response.

CHAPTER 5

CREDENTIALING AND TESTING REQUIREMENTS

"In the middle of difficulty lies opportunity."
Albert Einstein

KEY CONCEPTS

1. Credentialing indicates that an individual has met specified standards and is highly qualified to provide the specified service.
2. Certification, licensure, and registration are forms of credentialing.
3. State Departments of Education are responsible for credentialing schoolteachers.
4. The Praxis Series is the most commonly used national standardized teacher education test.
5. Non-teacher certifications are granted by a variety of organizations and agencies.

INTRODUCTION

Credentialing is a process whereby an individual meets the specified standards established by a credentialing body and is recognized for having done so. Credentialing documents that fact that practitioners are capable of providing quality service in the field in which they are certified. Professional associations, independent organizations and state governments administer credentialing. There are numerous benefits in credentialing professionals. These include:

- Documenting the individual's knowledge and skills in the field of practice

- Assisting employers to identify qualified professionals

- Assisting the public in recognizing the basic competencies of those who are credentialed

- Providing recognition to individual practitioners

- Recognizing a commitment to professional standards

- Strengthening professional preparation

- Facilitating geographic mobility of qualified practitioners.

- Requiring the individual to stay current in his/her profession

Credentialing may be through licensure, certification, or registration.

Licensure. Licensure is the generic term referring to all forms of agency or government (usually a state) grants of permission to individuals to practice a given profession. Licensure certifies that those licensed have attained specific standards of competence.

Certification. The U.S. Department of Health, Education, and Welfare define certification as "the process by which a nongovernmental agency or association grants recognition to an individual who has met certain predetermined qualifications. Such qualifications may include: (a) graduation from an accredited or approved program; (b) acceptable performance on a qualifying examination or series of examinations; and/or (c) completion of a given amount of work experience." Certification is a statement or document confirming completion of requirements in a specific field.

Registration. A less-restrictive form of state control is when states maintain a list of individuals through the process of registration. Registration is a process where the person's name is simply entered on a list and in some states registries of individuals are maintained by professional associations at the local level. The individual performs certain tasks, without requiring qualifications or passing an examination. This is seldom utilized in education.

Credentialing of Teachers

The No Child Left Behind Act of 2001 (Public Law 107-110) mandates that teachers in schools be highly qualified. State Departments of Education (SDE) are the credentialing agencies for the states and are responsible for ensuring that their teachers meet rigorous standards and are highly qualified. States must have a plan for achieving annual increases in the percentage of highly qualified teachers, to ensure that all teachers of core academic subjects are highly qualified by the 2005-2006 school year. A highly qualified teacher is defined by "No Child Left Behind" as:

- An elementary school teacher who:
  - Holds a bachelors degree
  - Has demonstrated mastery by passing a rigorous test in reading, writing, math and other areas of the curriculum

- A middle or high school teacher who:
  - Holds a bachelors degree
  - Has demonstrated competency in subject area taught by passing a rigorous state test, or through completion of an academic major, graduate degree, or comparable coursework.

Teacher certification is a process of legal recognition authorizing the individual holder of the certificate to perform specific services, usually teaching, in the public schools in the state. Initial teacher certification can be attained through traditional or alternative teacher certification programs. The traditional method of attaining certification is to complete a college degree program in teacher education that meets the state certification requirements. You must:

- Have a bachelor's degree from an accredited 4-year college or university.

- Complete teacher training through an approved teacher education program comprised of academic and professional curricula;

- Pass a national or state written basic skills test; and

- Pass the appropriate written teacher certification tests for the subject and grade level you will teach.

The National Center for Education Information reported, in a recent study entitled *Alternative Teacher Certification: A State-By-State Analysis 2002*, that more than 175,000 people have been certified through alternative routes. Thousands more are entering teaching through alternative preparation programs in colleges and universities. Currently, 45 out of 50 of the states offer some type of alternative certification program. This method of credentialing has become widely used as a result of teacher shortages and the lack of ethnic diversity among teachers in many areas. Alternative certification is a recent trend that allows persons who have content area competencies or who are from other career fields to obtain teaching credentials without going through a traditional teacher preparation program. The most common alternative certification programs:

- Have a strong academic coursework component;

- Allow candidates to go through programs in cohorts rather than as isolated individuals;

- Provide a qualified mentor to work with the candidate;

- Are field-based, allowing individuals to get into classrooms early in their preparation; and

- Are collaborative efforts involving state departments of education, institutions of higher education, and school districts.

There is any number of alternative paths to certification, all with varying programmatic characteristics. One example of requirements for an alternative certification program is listed below. The individual must:

- Hold a bachelors degree in the subject to be taught

- Achieve a passing score on a certification test

- Complete brief, intensive teacher training

- Complete a supervised teaching internship

- Be recommended for certification by the employing school district

Generally, initial teacher certification is issued for five years and must be renewed at five-year intervals thereafter. In order to renew certification, teachers must develop and implement a professional development plan. The plan may include college courses, and in-service and other workshops, seminars, and credits.

INTASC

INTASC's performance-based standards represent a core of teacher knowledge that transcends different disciplines, grade levels, and states. INTASC's standards provide information for beginning teachers about behaviors and expectations for performances.

According to INTASC standards, beginning teachers should have an understanding of the content they are teaching, the ability to work with diverse learners, and competency in a variety of instructional strategies. INTASC standards have helped shape teacher preparation programs as well as the licensing of teachers.

Teacher Education Testing Requirements

States vary in the number and types of minimum requirements that must be met by prospective teachers before they become certified to teach in the state. Many of the states require prospective teachers to pass a national standardized test, while other states require them to pass a state developed standardized test. Most states also require that prospective teachers take an additional certification test in their specialty area, such as health or physical education.

The most commonly used national standardized test is the Praxis Series tests. The Praxis Series: Professional Assessments for Beginning Teachers consists of validated assessments that provide accurate, reliable information for use by state education agencies in making licensing decisions. Colleges and universities may use the basic academic skills assessments to qualify individuals for entry into teacher education programs. The three categories of assessments in The Praxis Series correspond to the three milestones in teacher development: entering a teacher-training program, licensure for entering the profession, and the first year of teaching.

Praxis I: Academic Skills Assessments are designed to be taken early in a student's college career to measure reading, writing, and mathematics skills. The reading, writing, and mathematics assessments are available through either a paper-based or computer-based format.

Praxis II: Subject Assessments measure candidates' knowledge of the subjects they plan to teach as well as general and subject-specific pedagogical skills and knowledge. The pedagogy assessments, Principles of Learning and Teaching, are also included.

Praxis III: Classroom Performance Assessments are used to evaluate all aspects of a beginning teacher's practice and typically take place during the first year of teaching. These comprehensive assessments are designed to be conducted in the classroom by local assessors who employ nationally validated criteria to observe and evaluate a teacher's performance. Results are used to assist in making licensure decisions.

Many states have their own certification examinations. For example, Alabama requires prospective teachers to take the Alabama Prospective Teacher Test (APTT), California requires the California Basic Educational Skills Test (CBEST), Texas requires the Texas Examinations of Educator Standards (TExES). The TExES replaces the Examination for the Certification of Educators in Texas (ExCET) beginning in the 2002-2003 academic year. New York requires the New York State Teachers Certification Examination (NYTCE). Since state requirements vary from state to state, you should obtain requirements for each state by accessing the web site or directly contacting the State Department of Education.
In addition to the basic skills tests, prospective teachers are required, by most states, to pass a content specific test in the area in which you are planning to teach. This test may be a nationally or state developed examination.

TEACHER CERTIFICATIONS

The State Department of Education (SDE) certifies individuals in order to ensure that teachers are competent and are knowledgeable in the specific content area in which they will teach. Each state has unique certification requirements. Contact the SDE in the state in which you are interested in teaching for specific requirements for that state. Teacher certifications include:

- **Health Educator** (See Chapter 2)

- **Physical Educator** (See Chapter 3)

- **Adapted Physical Educator** (See Chapter 3)

NON-TEACHER CERTIFICATIONS

There are numerous state, district, and national associations/organizations that offer non-teacher certifications in the health, physical education related, and sports fields. A variety of certifications in health, physical education and sport will be discussed briefly and certifying agencies will be identified. Many of the certifications are applicable to health, physical education and sports. You are cautioned to be aware of the overabundance of "commercial certifications" available, especially in the fitness industry. Research certifications that you are considering in order to be sure that they are reputable certifications. Additional information concerning national certifications can be found by contacting your professional organizations, credentialing organizations, and or your campus Career Services Center.

Health Education Certifications

The emphasis placed on health education has become a focal point in our nation due to the *Healthy People 2010*, which has led to increased awareness of the need for effective health educators. The **National Commission for Health Education Credentialing, Inc.** (NCHEC) defines teacher educators as professionals who design, conduct and evaluate activities that help improve the health of all people. Health educators practice in a variety of settings that include schools, communities, health care facilities, businesses, colleges and government agencies. They may work with different populations: adults, the aged, children, and minorities. They are employed under a range of job titles such as patient educators, health education teachers, trainers, community organizers and health program managers. They may be process specialists: program planners, program implementers, program evaluators; or content specialists: HIV/AIDs, chronic diseases, injury or violence prevention, nutrition specialist. Health educators who work in the schools as health teachers are certified through the traditional or alternative certification process described in the previous section on credentialing of teachers and may also receive additional certifications in a variety of areas, as do other health educators. See Chapter 2 for more information on health careers.

Certified Health Education Specialists (CHES) Certification

The general certification for health educators is the Certified Health Education Specialist. CHESs are individuals come from a wide range of health education backgrounds. They have met the standards of competence established by NCHEC and have successfully passed the CHES examination. The CHES designation is an indication of professional competency and commitment to continued professional development. See the CHES Web site for responsibilities described in the NCHEC Framework. Eligibility to sit for the CHES examination is based on the following academic qualifications:

- A bachelor's, master's or doctoral degree from an accredited institution

- A major in health education, e.g., Health Education, Community Health Education, Public Health

- Or a minimum of 25 semester hours or 37 quarter hours of course work with specific preparation addressing the seven areas of responsibility.

National Commission for Health Education Credentialing, Inc.
944 Marcon Blvd. Suite 310
Allentown, PA   18109
(888) 624-3248 or (610) 264-8200
www.nchec.org

Health and Safety Certifications

The American Heart Association collaborates with schools, colleges and universities, and other organizations to promote health and wellness.   The organization specializes in cardiopulmonary resuscitation CPR, first aid, and aquatic certifications.

American Heart Association
7272 Greenville Ave.
Dallas, TX   75231-4596
(800) 242-8721
www.americanheart.org/

The **American Red Cross** has been the premiere provider of quality Health and Safety Training. The American Red Cross is committed to helping the community prevent, prepare for, and respond to emergencies at home, at work, and at play. Selected areas in which individuals may be certified are identified in Table 5.1.

American Red Cross (National Headquarters)
431 Eighteenth Street, NW
Washington, DC 20006
(202-737-8300)
www.redcross.org

Dieticians/Nutritionists Certifications

Dietetics is the high-tech science of applying food and nutrition to health. Dietetics/nutrition professionals work in education, healthcare, research, sales, marketing and public relations, government, restaurant management, fitness, food industry, and in private practice. The Commission on Accreditation for Dietetics Education (CADE) is the **American Dietetic Association**'s (ADA) accrediting agency for education program preparing students for careers as registered dietitians (RD) or dietetic technicians, registered (DTR). Selected information on all accredited/approved programs is published annually in the Directory of Dietetics Programs and the Web site.

American Dietetic Association
(800) 877-1600
www.eatright.org/nuresources.html

American College of Sport Medicine (ACSM) - refer to physical education and related area certifications.

The Cooper Institute for Aerobics Research - refer to physical education and related area certifications.

Table 5.1   Selected American Red Cross Certifications

American Red Cross Certifications	
Community CPR	Skills include how to give first aid for choking, other respiratory emergencies and CPR for adults, infants and children. This course is designed for individuals in the community who want to learn CPR skills for all ages
Standard First Aid	Trains individuals in the workplace and community to overcome any reluctance to act in emergency situations and to recognize and care for life-threatening emergencies such as respiratory or cardiac problems, sudden illness, and injury
Sports Safety Training	This course is designed to enable coaches and others to prevent, prepare for, and respond to sports related inquiries and emergencies
CPR for the Professional Rescuer (CPR-FPR)	Emphasizes the role of the professional rescuer in the EMS system, providing emergency care, recognizing and responding to respiratory and cardiac emergencies in infants, children and adults, and performing specialized skills and techniques used by professional rescuers
HIV/AIDS	Prepares you as an instructor to teach and present basic HIV/AIDS information. It will help you to feel comfortable talking about sensitive subjects and to be nonjudgmental and culturally sensitive to those with whom you talk. Prerequisite: ICT, Starter Facts and Facts Practice
Community First Aid and Safety Instructor	Instructor course, participants learn how to teach standard first aid, CPR, and community first aid and safety
Water Safety Instructor	Instructor candidates are trained in 36 hours to teach the Infant and Preschool Aquatics Program; the several levels of the Learn to Swim Program; the community Water Safety and Water Safety instructor Aide courses; and for eligible individuals, the Safety Training for Swim Coaches course. The minimum age is 17 by the end of the course and the certificate expires in two years

Physical Education and Related Area Certifications

There are numerous related careers in the area of physical education. These related careers include: fitness/health, recreation, therapy-related, and other related areas. Each related area generally encompasses a broad scope of careers in a wide variety of settings. The following section gives a sampling of areas requiring credentialing and some of the credentialing agencies. See Chapter 3 for more information on physical education related careers. Contact the credentialing agencies for more specific information on the credentialing process.

Fitness Trainers/Aerobics Instructors Certifications

Fitness trainer and aerobics instructor certification is available from many credentialing organizations. Most certifications require the individual to pass a written examination to test knowledge and a practical examination to assess skills. Certification is renewable at intervals specified by the credentialing organization. Continuing certification requires documentation of continuing education. See Table 6.2 for a brief description of selected certifications.

American College of Sports Medicine (ACSM)
401 West Michigan Street
Indianapolis, IN 46206-3233
(317) 637-9200
www.acsm.org
www.nata.org

Table 5.2 Selected fitness/health certifications

The ACSM offers Clinical Track and Fitness/Health Track Certifications	
Program Director	Highest level of ACSM certification for professionals in the Clinical Track; requires demonstration of competence in administration, design and implementation of safe and effective clinical exercise programs
Exercise Specialist	Cardiac rehabilitation certification; requires a wide range of clinical situations and patient-issues such as history-taking and assessment; counseling and education; activity and lifestyle modifications and emergency response
The Exercise Test Technologist	Certifies trained professionals who demonstrate knowledge, competence and skills required to deliver safe and valid exercise-related tests including a graded exercise test, electrocardiogram (ECG), pulmonary function test and oxygen uptake
Health and Fitness Director	Highest level of certification in the Health and Fitness Track; candidates must demonstrate administrative, supervisory, practical and theoretical competence in order to develop and manage preventive exercise and health-enhancement programs
Health/Fitness Instructor	Certifies those who can successfully lead exercise and health-enhancement programs; must also be able to show adequate knowledge of health appraisal techniques, risk factor identification and sub-maximal exercise testing; should demonstrate an understanding of the techniques for motivating, teaching, and counseling individuals to promote lifestyle changes
Exercise Leader	Entry level certification for the health/fitness professional involved in on-the-floor exercise leadership; uses hands-on techniques to teach and demonstrate safe and effective methods of exercise which apply the fundamental principles of exercise science; includes ability to implement exercise prescriptions developed by others and/or the field test results
Advance Personal Trainer	Certifies those with knowledge in nutrition, exercise programming, diagnostics, program management and techniques for working with special populations; designed for rehabilitation specialists, fitness instructors, and personal trainers

Aerobics and Fitness Association of America (AFAA)
15250 Ventura Boulevard, Suite 200
Sherman Oaks, CA 91403
(800) 446-2322

Table 5.3 **The Aerobics and Fitness Association of America (AFAA) Certifications**

The Aerobics and Fitness Association of America (AFAA) Certifications	
Fitness Practitioner	Advanced knowledge in nutrition, assessment, one-on-one training, and counseling for fitness management for life.
Personal Trainer/Fitness Counselor	Designed for fitness professionals who works individually in individualized fitness assessment and program design
Step Aerobics Instructor	Step aerobics course is designed to teach practical skills and knowledge in order to conduct safe, effective step aerobics classes
Advanced Personal Trainer	Designed for personal trainers or exercise science program graduates; includes information about lifting, spotting techniques, safety issues, and program design.

American Council on Exercise (ACE)
5820 Oberlin Drive, Suite 102
San Diego, CA 92121
(800) 825-3636

American Fitness Professionals & Associates (AFPA)
PO Box 214
Ship Bottom, NJ 08008
(609) 978-7583
www.afpafitness.com/main.htm

Exer-Safety Association
3785 West Commodore Cove
Reminderville, OH 44202
(216) 562-8280

National Dance-Exercise Instructor's Training Association
1503 S. Washington Avenue, Suite 208
Minneapolis, MN 55454
(800) 237-6242
www.ndeita.com

National Council of Strength & Fitness
1320 S. Dixie Hwy, Suite 910
Coral Gables, FL 33146
(800) 772-NCFS
www.NCSF.org

International Association of Fitness Professionals
6190 Cornerstone Court
East, Suite 204
San Diego, CA 92121-3773
(800) 999-4332

United States Water Fitness Association
P.O. Box 3279
Boynton Beach, FL 33424
(407) 732-9908

Fitness Research

The **Cooper Institute for Aerobics Research** has become widely acclaimed as one of the leaders in preventive medicine research and education. The Cooper Institute conducts research in epidemiology, exercise physiology, behavior change, hypertension, children's health issues, obesity, nutrition, aging, and other health issues. Training and certification programs for fitness leaders and health professionals are conducted annually on the Dallas campus and at other sites throughout the United States.

The Cooper Institute for Aerobics Research
12330 Preston Road
Dallas, TX 75230
(972) 341-3200
(800) 635-7050
www.cooperinst.org/

Table 5.4   Selected Cooper Institute for Aerobics Research Certifications

The Cooper Institute for Aerobics Research Certifications	
Physical Fitness Specialist (Personal Trainer)	Instruction in screening options, fitness assessment and goal setting, exercise prescriptions, nutritional programs, motivational techniques, feedback methods, safety programming, exercise physiology, anatomy, kinesiology, and wellness and coronary risk; designed for personal trainers or fitness instructors in health and fitness center, clubs, and clinics; certification requires passing scores on both written and practicum examination and current CPR certification is required
Master Fitness Specialist	Certification built on knowledge learned during a previous certification program; includes in-depth, research-based information on stress management, cholesterol update, medications and CHD, low back health, controversial exercises, ergogenic aids and athletic performance, sports nutrition, stress testing, body composition assessment, physiology of aging, resting metabolic rate, and behavior change; requires passing scores on both written and practicum examination; current CPR certification is required
Biomechanics of Resistance Training Specialty Certification	Content includes anatomy and kinesiology overview, training for the upper body, training for the lower body, training for the core body, proper mechanics, spotting techniques, program designed for resistive exercise and business empowerment for success; requires passing scores on both written and practicum examinations; current CPR certification is required
Group Exercise Leadership	Develops basic level leadership and technical skills for conducting group exercise programs; designed for exercise and aerobics instructors who are already teaching or entering the profession; content includes scripting class, leadership/teaching techniques, exercise choreography, rhythmical skills and techniques, proper body alignment, safety programming, motivation strategies, scientific foundations, and program planning
Health Promotion Director	Provides training in starting or revitalizing a health promotion program, leadership, supervision and administrative skills using case studies and the implementation of activities that enhance and support healthful behavior changes, and is designed for experience health promotion professionals
Aquatics Specialty	Lectures and activity sessions on aquatic exercise, safety, special populations, equipment, proto-type lessons, and deep water walking; designed for aerobic instructors, personal trainers, and other health and fitness professionals who work with people who exercise in the water

SPORT/COACHING CERTIFICATIONS

The **National Association for Sport and Physical Education** developed *National Standards for Athletic Coaches* to provide a national framework for organizations and agencies that provide coaching education and training. These standards are not a coaching certification program but a framework for the education of coaches. Knowledge, skills, and values are associated with effective and appropriate coaching of athletes. The standards are organized into 37 standards, grouped into 8 domains. The 8 domains and standards associated with each domain are:

- Injuries: Prevention, Care, and Management
- Risk Management
- Growth, Development, and Learning
- Training, Conditioning, and Nutrition
- Social/Psychological Aspects of Coaching
- Skills, Tactics, and Strategies
- Teaching and Coaching
- Professional Preparation and Development

National Association for Sport and Physical Education
1900 Association Dr.
Reston, VA 22091
(703) 476-3417
www.aahperd.org/naspe/athstds.html

Athletic Training Certifications

The **National Athletic Trainers Association Board of Certification** (NATABOC) provides a certification program for entry-level athletic trainers and recertification standards for certified athletic trainers. The purpose of the entry-level certification program is to establish standards for entry into the profession of athletic training. A continuing education requirement is established so that a certified athletic trainer must satisfy in order to maintain status as an NATABOC certified athletic trainer. The mission of the NATA BOC is: to certify athletic trainers and to identify for the public, quality healthcare professionals through a system of certification, adjudication, standards of practice and continuing competency programs.

National Athletic Trainers Association
2952 Stemmons Freeway, Suite 200
Dallas, TX 75247-6196
(214) 637-6282 or (800) TRY-NATA
www.nata.org

Strength and Conditioning Certifications

The **National Strength and Conditioning Association** (NSCA) is the professional membership organization of persons involved in the conditioning of athletes. Members who support the Association make a firm commitment to the organizations motto: An optimum athletic performance through total conditioning.

National Strength and Conditioning Association
1955 North Union Blvd.
Colorado Springs, CO 80909
(719) 632-6722
www.nsca-lift.org

Youth Sports Certifications

The **American Sport Education Program (ASEP)** is the most widely used coaching education   program in the United States. Educational programs are designed for sport coaches, sport directors and   sport   parents. ASEP provides training in coaching the young athlete, coaching principles, sports drugs, first aid, teaching sports skills and a variety of sport sciences. ASEP provides education at three levels:

- Volunteer level primarily for youth sport coaches
- Leader level for leaders of scholastic and club sports
- Master level for those who aspire to higher level of competency.

American Sport Education Program
P.O. Box 5076
Champaign, IL   61825-5076
(800) 747-4457
www.asep.com/

The **National Alliance Youth Sports Coaches Association (NYSCA)** is a national training system for volunteer sports youth coaches. Coaches must participate in a 3-year, 3-level program to qualify for certification. The three year training levels include:

- First year training emphasizes the development approach to coaching and safety
- Second year focuses on physiological and psychological issues
- Third year features sport techniques

The National Alliance for Youth Sports
2050 Vista Parkway
W. Palm Beach, FL   33411-2718
(800) 729-2057
www.nays.org

National Federation of High School Associations (NFHSA)
11724 NW Plaza Circle
P.O. Box 20626
Kansas City, MO 64195-0626
(816) 464-5400

National Intramural-Recreational Sports Association (NIRSA)
850 S.W. 15th St.
Corvalis, OR 97333-4145
(541) 737-2088

National Recreation and Park Association (NRPA)
2237 Belmont Ridge Road
Ashburn, VA 20148
(703) 858-2162
www.nrpa.org

Sports Officials Certifications

The growth in all types of sports programs has created a need for sports officials on all levels. Sports officials usually begin their officiating career as a part-time job, but many individuals pursue it on a full time basis. Certification requires passing a written and a practical examination. Beginning official must spend a given number of hours working with an experiences official before working alone.

National Amateur Baseball Association
P. O. Box 705
12406 Keynote Lane
Bowie, MD   20715
(301) 262-0770

National Association of Sports Officials (NASO)
2017 Latherop Ave.
Rcine, WI   35405
(414) 632-5448

 National Federation of State High School Associations (NFIOA)
11724 N. W. Plaza Circle
P. O. Box 20626
Kansas City, MO   64195-0626
(816) 464-5400

National Youth Sports Association (NYSA)
2050 Vista Parkway
West Palm Beach, FL   33411-2718
(800) 729-2057

United States Tennis Association (USTA)
70 W. Red Oak Lane
White Plains, NY   10604
(914) 696-7000

SUMMARY

Certification in health, physical education and sport doesn't have to be an impossible dream. Narrowing your choices of certifications may eliminate certain opportunities for you, which is why it is important that you gain a variety of hands-on experiences and attain broad based knowledge and skills.

Teacher preparation in health, physical education and sport does not end upon receipt of a diploma and a teacher's certificate. Begin preparing academically and learning about specific certification and testing requirements early in your professional studies. Individuals must continue to educate themselves by taking graduate courses in specific content areas or in advanced teaching methods, joining local, state, regional, and national health, physical education and sport professional organizations and attending professional conferences. It is extremely valuable to continue reading up-to-date textbooks, journals, periodicals and other professional publications and attending in-service workshops that deal with related topics. In addition, seek out experiences, internships in teaching, health, physical education and sport related activities.

Take the time now to reflect upon your talents, goals, experience, professional training, professional involvement and the types of certifications needed in order to attain your choice in a career. Remember that proper academic preparation and effective communication are important keys to your career. Be yourself, think positive and keep doing what you need to do to win and achieve your goals. Realize that you are exchanging a part of your life, for the time you spend now, in search of a career to fulfill your life's dream.

REFLECTIONS

1. Research the teacher certification requirements in each state that touches the border of your home state. Compare the requirements from one of the states with those in the state where you currently live. Use Laboratory 6.1 for your response.

2. Access the AAHPERD Web site and read the National Standards for Athletic Coaches. Reflect on your own athletic experiences and compare the actions and behaviors of your coaches to the standards. Did your coaches meet these standards? What were their weaknesses? Discuss the importance of these standards for coaches in your class.

WEBSITES

www.acsm.org
American College of Sports Medicine

www.sbcoe.k12.ca.us/testingR.html
Education Testing and Standards

www.nata.org
National Athletic Trainers Association

www.ed.gov/nclb/landing.jhml
No Child Left Behind

www.ets.org/portal/site/ets/menuitem.tab
Praxis Series

www.isbe.state.il.us/research/portal/standards.htm
Standards/Assessment/Accountability

www.eduhound.com/k12statetesting.cfm
U.S. Dept. of Education: State Comprehensive Testing, Accountability and Assessment

BIBLIOGRAPHY

American Alliance for Health, Physical Education, Recreation and Dance. (1999*). Resolution: Teacher Professional Preparation in Health Education.* www.aahperd.org/aahe/programs-hivresolution.html

American Red Cross. www.redcross.org

Anspaugh, D.J. and Ezell, G. (2007). *Teaching Today's Health,* 8th ed. Boston: MA: Pearson Education.

Girvan, J.T.; McKenzie, J.F.; and Cottnell, R.R. (2005). *Principles & Foundations of Health Promotion and Education*, 3rd ed. Boston, MA: Pearson Education.

Interstate New Teacher Assessment and Support Consortium Standards. http://www.ccsso.org/content/pdfs/corestrd.pdf.

Lumpkin, A. (2007). *Introduction to Physical Education, Exercise Science, and Sport Studies,* 7th ed. Boston, MA: McGraw-Hill.

National Association for Sport and Physical Education. *National Standards for Athletic Coaches, 1994.* American Alliance for Health, Physical Education, Recreation and Dance.

The Praxis Series: Professional Assessments for Beginning Teachers. www.ets.org/praxis/index.html

U. S. Department of Education. (2002). *Meeting the Highly Qualified Teachers Challenge: The Secretary's Annual Report of Teacher Quality.* Washington, D. C.

Wuest, D.A. and Bucher, C.A. (2006). *Foundations of Physical Education, Exercise Science, and Sport*, 15th ed. Boston, MA: McGraw-Hill.

LABORATORY ACTIVITY 5.1

NAME _____ DATE _____

COURSE _____ SECTION _____

Research the teacher certification requirements in each state that touches the border of your home state. Compare the requirements from one of the states with those in the state where you currently live, or would like to live.

Home state:

Adjoining states:

Comparison:

LABORATORY ACTIVITY 5.2

NAME _____ DATE _____

COURSE _____ SECTION _____

Using the Web sites provided in this chapter, find the testing site in your state where you can take the certified health, physical education, and coaching examination.

CHAPTER 6

WRITING YOUR RESUME

"The purpose of a resume is to get you the job interview; the interview gets you the job."
Anonymous

KEY CONCEPTS

1. The three R's in resume writing include research the school/organization, research the position, and research yourself.
2. The three basic types of resumes include the chronological resume, functional resume, and the chronological/functional resume.
3. The cover letter is a personalized letter that is your first opportunity to introduce yourself, present your qualifications and show the search committee that you are a potential candidate for the position.
4. There are seven basic types of letters.

INTRODUCTION

Before you finish college, you will need to develop your own customized resume. Designing your resume is a necessity for most all jobs whether it is for an internship, part-time job, a teacher, CEO, health or sports professional. You must carefully and objectively examine this document before sending it to your potential employer, if not, most likely, it will be thrown in the trash. Resume readers will view your resume on an average of 15-20 seconds. Read the advertisements; determine if you have the right credentials and apply for those for which you are qualified. To obtain the professional career you desire the following information on resume writing will provide you with a guide to the appropriate sources.

The resume must quickly show your accomplishments and skills and attract the reader's attention. You only get one brief chance – so your resume must represent your best effort.

RESUME WRITING

Developing an effective resume is an important aspect between employment and unemployment. Not all resumes need to look the same. Different people need to emphasize things in different ways. The three R's, which must be considered in resume writing, are research, research, and research. You must know what the prospective school/organization does, what the position entails, and whether you have the qualifications, before submitting your resume. In other words, you must do research about the school/organization, the position and about the type of employee that is needed.

Research the School/Organization

In researching the school/organization read literature the school/organization has in career libraries, use the information highway, Internet or call the school district/organization. Find out the name of the supervisor and give him/her a call. Ask if there are openings in your field, explain that you are trying to decide whether to apply to their school/organization, ask for recommendations for the next steps, thank the person for the information, and ask to whom your resume should be directed.

Research the Position

The more you know about the position, the better you will be in selling yourself and to write your resume to that position. Seek to interview someone who does the same job. Ask questions such as: what kind of turnover the department experiences, what they like about the position and the company, what they dislike about it, and whether they value education over experience (or vice versa).

Research Yourself

Certain information is needed to evaluate your qualifications and determine if you meet the requirements necessary in obtaining a job. If your resume or application does not provide all the information requested in the job vacancy announcement, you may lose consideration for the job. Speed the selection process by keeping your resume or application brief and sending only the requested material.

Your goal is to get the job that you will enjoy. As a health, physical education and sports practitioner/professional is this the type of job you really want? Odds are that you will not hold this position for more than two or three years so it is not a career commitment. However two or three years are an eternity in spending in a job you do not like. Before going to the interview, review the resume that you submitted to this particular employer.

The key components of a resume include the format, appearance, length, and content. The format chosen will depend on the job you wish to obtain, in this case a teaching, health or sport related career. Appearance often determines if the resume is reviewed so it should be concise and organized. Your resume should be completed on a word-processor and professionally copied with high quality white paper or off-white paper. There must be no typographical errors. The length of the resume will vary; usually a one-page resume works well for recent graduates and an individual with extensive work experience will require two pages. Limit information to what is pertinent to the current job objective. The content of the resume should have a clear objective with the information presented relative to the objective. Information should be included in descending order of importance. Remember, the purpose of a resume is to get the interview; the interview gets you the job.

Cover Letters

Your cover letter is a personalized letter that is your first opportunity to introduce yourself, present your qualifications and show the search committee that you are a potential candidate for the position. It presents your intentions, availability and indicates that you are serious about your job search. A cover letter must entice the reader to consider you amidst hundreds or even thousands of candidates for any one job opening.

The cover letter should be clear and to the point including the specific job title for which you are applying and two to three reasons why your experience is good for this position. It includes a brief outline of your career highlights, provides facts, list relevant skills and state accomplishments on recent jobs that will be impressive. Use the following suggestions to write your cover letter.

- Personalize it to the organization. Find out whom to write to as it differs with various careers. If you were seeking a marketing position at an advertising agency, you would write to the director of account services. Some organizations you would write to the director of human resources for the entire organization. Never write "To whom it may concern." References in the career library, the Internet can help you and so can your academic advisor.
- State the reason for your interest in the organization. Show that you have done your homework by mentioning organization specifics and address the cover letter to a specific individual whenever possible.
- State your intentions and qualification up front. Make sure they understand why you are sending your resume.
- Tell what makes you different? Highlight your strengths. Emphasize your talents, experiences and your skills to show that you would be a valuable addition to the team. Also, briefly include volunteer or professional experience.
- Do not include negative information. Never include conflicts with previous employers, pending litigation suits or sarcastic remarks.
- Be direct! Clean, error-free presentation, combined with strong phrasing and solid facts will encourage the reader to review the attached resume and call you in for an interview.
- Do not include salary or relocation information. If a prospective employer requests it, include it. For example, you could write: "My salary requirements are $50,000-$60,000 (negotiable)." Or you might write: "My current salary is $52,000 at ABC organization." Eliminating this information from your cover letter may justify your resume getting tossed out. Never include salary and relocation information on your resume.
- Take action steps. Use a proactive approach in your cover letter. State the fact that you are available for a personal interview; give your home, work, email and/or cell phone numbers where you can be reached; note that you will follow up by phone to provide any additional information required.

Figure 6.1 Cover Letter

Milton E. Wilson
5060 Charleston Way
Greenville, NC 25069

May 24, 2008

Mike E. Jones
VP, Sales and Marketing
Health Southeast Supplier
4002 Frontier Lane
Montgomery, AL 36072

Dear Mr. Jones:

When I receive my B.A. degree this spring, I would very much like to begin a career as a health supplier salesperson. I had no idea I would be interested in this career when I majored in communications. Then I chose a minor in health and discovered they fit so closely together. In addition, I have a friend who works for a health company in my city in sales of health supplies. I have spent a good deal of time with him, shadowed him on sales calls, and decided this was the career I wanted to pursue.

I plan to visit Montgomery sometime around August 10 and would greatly appreciate a few moments of your time. If you have no openings at your company, perhaps you might refer me to other companies involved in health supplies. I will call you at least a week before I make my trip to see if you have time to visit with me.

Sincerely,

(signature)

Lori Abbot

TYPES OF RESUMES

Three types of resumes are discussed in this section. These include the chronological, functional and the combination of the chronological/functional resume. Use the type of resume that best suits your career objectives.

Chronological Resume

A chronological resume presents your education and work experience in a straightforward, reverse chronological order. If the majority of your work experience is related to your stated job objective, the chronological style can be effective.

Functional or Skills Resume

A functional or skills resume differs from a chronological resume by concentrating on skills that you have used that relate to your stated objective rather than on the job you have had. A functional/skills resume is effective if your work experience has not been closely related to your job objective, if you are changing careers, or if you are seeking a promotion. In this format you elaborate on the skills necessary to perform the desired job and how you have demonstrated those same skills in a different type of job.

Chronological/Functional Resume

A chronological/functional resume is the combination of the chronological and functional resume, which uses elements of both styles. The skills section (also called qualifications) identifies your skills in relation to your job objective, but does not elaborate on your experiences or accomplishments for each skill mentioned. This format can be effective if at least some of your work experience is related to your job objective and you want to outline some highlights of your work.

RESUME CONTENT

Your resume or application should contain the following categories. These are suggestions: adopt those categories that best fit your career objective.

- **Job information.** Announcement number, and title and grade(s) of the job for which you are applying.
- **Personal data.** Full name, mailing address (with ZIP Code) day/evening phone numbers (with area code) Your name should be the most obvious piece of information. Provide an e-mail address if applicable.
- **Keyword skills, if appropriate.** Usually just below the objective or below education. Keyword skills are like a table of contents or an outline, which you are saying, "I am going to tell you more in the experience section." See Figure 6.3.

General Guidelines for Resumes

- Limit resume to one page or if you have an extensive employment history no more than two pages. Limit your information to what is important to their job objective. Place the most important information on the first page if you elect to submit a two-page resume.
- Make sure the format is well organized and concise. An organized resume determines whether a resume is read.
- Use white or off-white high quality paper.
- Always type or word-process your resume and have it professionally copied.
- Make sure the resume is free of misspelled words, typographical errors, and grammatical errors. Handwritten information is unacceptable.
- Have a friend or professional edit your resume.
- Design the resume with a specific objective. Present information important to the objective first.
- List information in descending order of importance.
- Be selective about the information you include in resume.
- Never exaggerate or falsify information.
- Sell yourself. Attract attention to your special qualities.
- Concentrate on the positive and use action words to highlight your personal traits (See Table 6.1 Action Words).

Figure 6.2 CHRONOLOGICAL RESUME: Format and Content Description

---

NAME
Email address

Local Address   Permanent Address
City, State, ZIP   City, State, ZIP
Phone Number w/Area Code   Phone Number w/Area Code

OBJECTIVE:
    Be specific

EDUCATION:
    List most recent degree first, major, institution and date of graduation or expected graduation. Point out areas of specialization in academic work, honors.

    If applicable, include:
    Thesis Title
    Faculty Research Advisor
    Publications

    You may wish to add an addendum that identifies the courses you have taken, grouped into two or three meaningful categories.

RELATED EXPERIENCE:
    Your job title, name of organization, description of your duties, including the variety of assignments, amount of responsibility, number of people supervised, and special accomplishments, dates. Include military service if applicable.

EXTRACURRICULAR/LEADERSHIP
    Job title, name of organization, brief (optional) description of responsibilities, and dates.

INTERESTS (Optional Category)

REFERENCES
    Write "Available upon request" or "References attached"
    On a separate page, give names, titles, business mailing addresses and telephone numbers of two or three business references. Do not use relatives, friends, or other students as references.

Figure 6.3 FUNCTIONAL/SKILLS RESUME: Format and Content Description

---

NAME
Email address

Local Address	Permanent Address
City, State, ZIP	City, State, ZIP
Phone Number w/Area Code	Phone Number w/Area Code

OBJECTIVE:
> Be specific

EDUCATION:
> List most recent degree first, major, institution and date of graduation. Honors, if applicable, and if you feel they are important.

KEYWORD SKILLS:
> In this section, isolate three to five of your strongest demonstrated skills. The skills you select should be essential to the type of job you have identified in your objective. For each skill you have chosen summarize your accomplishments and experiences that pertain. You need not mention the specific job in this section, as you will do so in the "Employment History" section. Be specific in discussing how you demonstrated your skills and, whenever possible, concentrate on the results you achieved in using the particular skills.
> For example: Initiative, Organization, Supervision, Computer

EXPERIENCE
> Job title, employer, duties, and dates.

ACTIVITIES/LEADERSHIP (Honors)
> Job title, name of organization, brief (optional) description of responsibilities and dates.

INTERESTS (Optional category)

REFERENCES
> Write "Available upon request" or "References attached"
> On a separate page, give names, titles, business mailing addresses and telephone numbers of two or three business references. Do not use relatives, friends, or other students as references.

Figure 6.4   COMBINATION CHRONOLOGICAL/FUNCTIONAL RESUME: Format and Content Description

---

NAME
Email address

Local Address   Permanent Address
City, State, ZIP   City, State, ZIP
Phone Number w/Area Code   Phone Number w/Area Code

OBJECTIVE:
    Be specific about the type of position desired.

SKILLS:
    In a list or brief paragraph, summarize three to five skills you have that related to your stated job objective. You should be able to utilize these skills with little or no supervision.

EDUCATION:
    Beginning with your most advanced degree, list degree, major, institution, date of graduation, and honors, if applicable.

RELATED COURSE WORK:
    (Optional category)

EXPERIENCE:
    List your job title, the organization for which you worked and a brief description of your duties, including the variety of tasks, type of responsibility, and any special accomplishments. Dates follow last.

INTERESTS:
    (Optional category)

REFERENCES
    Write "Available upon request" or "References attached"
    On a separate page, give names, titles, business mailing addresses and telephone numbers of two or three business references. Do not use relatives, friends, or other students as references.

Keyword Skills

Choose nouns that indicate your accomplishments rather than verbs that focus on duties. The keyword in an electronic resume should be organized into two sections. These include Keyword Preface and the main body of the resume. The Keyword Preface or Summary appears directly beneath your name and contact information at the top of your resume. It is an inventory of your most important assets. It runs about 20 to 30 items and each item is capitalized and ends with a period. Three points should be used in selecting your items:

- Your particular skills, abilities and competencies;
- Your experience using those skills, abilities and competencies; and
- Your accomplishments in using those skills, abilities and competencies on-the-job.

It is important to alter your resume to fit a particular job. Use key words in job posting and advertisements and include them in your resume. Electronically transmitted cover letters should include keywords.

Table 6.1   Action Words

achieved	dependable	led	reliable
adaptable	diagnosed	located	self-confident
assertive	determined	lifted	resilient
advertised	developed	listened	resourceful
aided	designed	learned	projected
allocated	diligent	lectured	published
approved	diplomatic	logical	ranked
arranged	disciplined	loyal	receptive
assisted	discreet	made	self-motivated
authored	documented	maintained	self-reliant
briefed	drafted	managed	sensitive sharp
broadminded	edited	mastered	sincere strong
brought	efficient	mature	studied
budgeted	effective	maximized	successful
built	energetic	mentored	supervised
charged	enterprising	modeled	supported
chartered	enthusiastic	modified	surveyed
classified	evaluated	monitored	tactful
checked	examined	objective	taught
committed	exceptional	open minded	tenacious
competent	experienced	outgoing	trained
conscientious	fair	participated	translated
creative	firm	personable	upgraded
cooperative	forceful honest	pleasant	utilized
debated	independent	poised	verified
decided	innovative	positive	visualized
dedicated	instrumental	practical	won
defined	judged	prepared	wrote
delegated	kept	productive	
delivered	launched	programmed	

Scanner-Friendly Resume

Filling your resume with key words may be the secret in getting the job. A large number of organizations use personnel search firms and are using the scanning technology. A computer checks databases for resumes that include these keywords. You will need a log of keywords that apply to your career and jot down the words as you come across them in magazines, class notes, newspaper ads, professional organization networking, etc.

Guidelines for Preparing a Scannable Resume

The easiest resumes to read and scan are resumes presented in a chronological order, such as to list and describe up to four jobs in order by date. In addition resumes should describe achievements rather than job titles and use combinations of resume types. The most difficult resumes to read and scan include resumes done in a newsletter layout, with adjusted spacing, large font sizes, graphics or line, too light of type print, paper which is too dark, script writing and those done on marble or heavy paper. The following guidelines apply when completing a scannable resume:

- Select keywords and arrange them in order of importance. List the names of software you use such as Microsoft Word and Lotus 1.2.3
- Use standard typefaces such as Times New Roman or Courier.

- Use font size between 10 and 14 points.
- Place name at the top of the page and use standard address format below your name. Name can be first text on page two. List address and each phone number on its own line.
- Use 8 1/2" x 11" white paper printed on one side only
- Use a 24-pin letter-quality or laser printer. Avoid low quality copies.
- Avoid graphics, pictures and gray screens (shading).
- Avoid or use horizontal and vertical lines sparingly and allow 1/4" of white space around them. Omit parentheses, brackets and boxes.
- Avoid fancy treatments such as italics, underline, shadows, and reverses (white letters on black background).
- When faxing a resume, set the fax machine on "fine mode" rather than "standard mode."
- Boldface type is acceptable, and /or all capital letters for section headings as long as the letters do not touch each other.
- Best paper weight for an electronic resume is copy grade (20lb.) or slightly heavier, such as offset printing grade (60 lb.).
- Never condense spacing between letters.
- Avoid two-column format or resumes that look like newspapers or newsletters.
- Avoid stapling or folding the resume. Send it flat in a large envelop.
- Use a maximum of two pages (one page preferred).
- Use jargon and acronyms specific to your career (spell out the acronyms).
- Use common headings such as Objective, Experience, Education, Professional Affiliations, Licenses, etc.

Sending Resumes by E-mail

When corresponding with a perspective employer for the first time, should you send your resume by e-mail? Before you make that decision, there are some things you need to know. First, you need to find out the company's policy or preference. Then, you need to be sure to prepare the resume properly.

You can begin by reviewing the job posting for application instructions. Most likely all the information you need can be found on the company's website. Review how the company would like you to apply and carefully follow the directions. If you don't follow the directions precisely, your application may not be considered.

The resume that you prepare to send electronically will contain the same information that you would include on a hard copy; however, you will need to adjust the format of your resume to make it easy for you to make revisions, post, and e-mail. A properly prepared resume will contain all of the necessary keywords to attract attention whether it is being scanned into a resume system, indexed and searched online, or read in hard copy.

When preparing your resume for e-mailing to employers it will need to be in a specific format. Formatting is important because it will prevent problems with jumbling and readability when it reaches the reader's inbox. Preparing your resume for e-mail is a simple process. For e-mail, the plain text version of ASCII resume is recommended.

A plain text resume is basically exactly what its called. It is free of formatting enhancements such as bold, underline, or fancy fonts. It will not be very attractive; however, it will be universally compatible, allowing you to control its appearance. This version of the resume is a text only document that can readily be copied or cut and pasted into the body of your e-mail and into on-line application forms. In addition, you will need to send a cover letter in the same e-mail. It is usually best to begin the e-mail with the cover letter. You should mention in the letter that your resume is included in the e-mail and then put your resume within the e-mail. A brief description of how to set up your plain text version resume is shown below.

1. Set your margins so that you have 6.5 inches of text displayed. This will not allow your text from rolling onto the next line.
2. Use a 12-point font such as Courier or Times New Roman.
3. If you must change it up, use asterisks, O's, plusses, etc. without fearing that they will be converted into questions marks, as may happen with bullets.

As many as 80% of employers accept resumes and applications online. In addition, there are hundreds of sites where you can post your resume online and complete an online job application. Some sites let you upload an existing resume with the click of a button. On other sites, you can cut and paste or use a resume builder. Once you have uploaded your resume, you will be able to search for jobs that interest you, and submit your application or resume with ease.

International Resumes

Most international job applicants submit many copies of one generic resume to anyone receiving resumes, without any customization or understanding of the prospective employer. This strategy rarely works and is even less effective for international applicants. Unless you have specific technical skills for which you know an employer is looking, don't waste your time applying for these jobs. Blanketing the universe electronically without real contacts in organizations most likely will not work.

AVOIDING THE DANGERS IN RESUME WRITING

- **Appearances.** Use good quality paper, check for typos, grammatical errors and stains. Use the spell-check and ask a friend to review the resume to find mistakes.

- **Too long.** Resumes should be one page and if your career warrants a two-page, create a document that reflects the full range of your accomplishments and experiences. Don't reduce the type size that your resume becomes difficult to read. If you need assistance to complete the resume ask a career center professional.

- **Grammatical, spelling or typographical errors.** Errors suggest poor education, lack of intelligence and carelessness. Don't rely on spell-checkers or grammar-checkers on the computer. Solicit a minimum of two other proofreaders before submitting.

- **Too sparse.** Provide more than the bare essentials, especially when describing related work experience, skills, activities, interests, etc. Include professional memberships.

- **Hard to read.** A copied or poorly typed resume looks unprofessional. Use a computer, plain typeface, and 10-14 font. Asterisks, bullets, underlining, boldface type and italics should be used only to make the document easier to read. Ask for professional assistance.

- **Too verbose.** Using too many words to say too little. Be careful using jargon and use only if it is specific to your career and avoid slang. Say as much as possible with a few words. A, an, and the can almost always be left out.

- **Irrelevant information.** Customize each resume to each position you seek. Always include education and relevant work experience such as skills, accomplishments, activities and hobbies. Do not include marital status, age, sex, children, height, weight, health, religious preference, etc.

- **Too generic.** Apply for the position advertised, not just any job or position.

- **Boring.** Resume should be dynamic. Begin every statement with an action verb. Use active verbs, describing what you accomplished on the job. Avoid repeating words, especially the first word in a section.

- **Use quality bond paper.** Organizations are scanning resumes into a database, so use white paper, black ink, plain type and avoid symbols, underlining or italics.

- **Sell you.** Put your best qualities forward without misrepresentation, arrogance, or falsification.

- **No extra papers.** Don't include copies of transcripts, awards, letters of recommendation, unless you are specifically asked to do so. If you are called in for an interview, bring these extra materials along in your briefcase to show-and-tell.

- **No personal information.** Personal information does not belong on a resume. Do not include information on your age, ethnicity, family, or marital status.

WHEN TO UPDATE YOUR RESUME

- Time flies… your resume does not include the past year of your accomplishments and work at your present job.

- No Personal items… no personal information should be in your resume.

- Address/telephone numbers… information is still listed at your last home/telephone number.

- Technology update… resume does not list computer software you have learned within the last two years.

- Job Accomplishments… your last resume lists more fraternity, awards and college sports than your present job accomplishments.

- Career… your old resume lists your previous jobs even though you have been in your present job for four years.

- New Job… an opportunity for a new job but you must have your resume to the prospective employer by the next day.

- Do you know where to find the current version of your resume on your hard drive?

- Organization layoffs… rumors of layoffs are circulating. Is your current resume updated ready to seek another job opportunity?

SUMMARY

Resume writing is the first step to securing a job in your desired profession. Knowing the types of resumes and how to compose them will make the job search process easier. Having the general guidelines of appearance, objectives, certain dos and don'ts will tremendously improve your chances of getting that interview of a lifetime.

REFLECTIONS

1. Identify and discuss the three types of resumes. Select one type and compose a one page resume. Use Laboratory 6. 1 for your response.

2. Using the internet, construct an on-line resume. Use Laboratory 6.2 for your response.

WEB SITES

www.10minuteresume.com/
Resume Writing

www.jobsmart.org/tools/resume/index.cfm
JobStarresumes & Cover Letters

www.provenresumes.com/
Resume Writing Tips

www.rileyguide.com/eresume.html
Prepare Your Resume for E-mail and Online Posting

BIBLIOGRAPHY

Floyd, P. and Allen, B. (2008). *Professional Preparation of Pre-Service Teachers*. Boston, MA: Pearson Education.

Developing a Winning Resume, Career Services Center. Alabama State University.

In Search of the Perfect Resume, Career Services Center. Alabama State University.

Ryan, Robin (2005). *21 Ways to Improve Your Resume*. www.robinryan.com.

Ryan, Robin (2008). *Winning Resumes*, 2nd ed. John Wiley & Sons. www.robinryan.com.

Ryan, Robin (2008). *Winning Cover Letters*, 2nd ed. John Wiley & Sons. www.robinryan.com.

Wuest, D.A. and Bucher, C. (2006). *Foundations of Physical Education, Exercise Science, and Sport*, 15th ed. Boston, MA: WCB/McGraw-Hill.

LABORATORY ACTIVITY 6.1

NAME _____ DATE _____

COURSE _____ SECTION _____

Identify and discuss the three types of resumes and compose a one page resume for one type. Use this Lab to write your resume.

LABORATORY ACTIVITY 6.2

NAME _____ DATE _____

COURSE _____ SECTION _____

Using the information and web features provided in this chapter, construct an on-line resume. Discuss this resume with your instructor for feedback. Record your results below.

CHAPTER 7

PRESENTING A POSITIVE IMAGE

"Put yourself in the driver's seat to reach your destination"
Robert Orndorff

KEY CONCEPTS

1. There are different types of interviews.
2. Employers have expectations of prospective employees.
3. The typical structure of the interview consists of three phases: before, during, and after.
4. There are seven steps to effective preparation for the interview.
5. Communication is a key element in interviewing.
6. Dressing for success is essential for a successful interview.
7. It is necessary to evaluate an offer before you accept the position.

INTRODUCTION

Now that you have made a good impression with your resume, it is time for the interview. The purpose of the interview is to narrow the list of potential candidates until the most qualified candidate in the opinion if the interviewer(s) is found, which does not necessarily mean the one who may be the "most qualified" on paper. If you want to be hired be prepared to sell yourself as the best person for the position.

TYPES OF INTERVIEWS

Employers often use a variety of types of interviews to determine your capabilities. It is to your advantage to be well prepared for a variety of possible interview situations. The following are common types of interviews and suggestions on how to be successful in each situation.

Information/Networking Interview

An information/networking interview is one of the most powerful job search strategies in seeking employment. This type interview is an exeellent way to obtain information regarding different types of specialty areas or careers, discuss major issues in selected careers, gain pertinent information about careers of interest, secure names of contacts and future job references. Once you identify what you do well and what you enjoy doing, talk with people working in your area of interest. Such interviews yield valuable information about careers, particularly the skills and experiences employers expect you to have.

Prepare a list of questions to ask and your resume to hand out to potential employers. Some suggested questions you may ask during these interviews are:

- What are the major responsibilities of your career?
- What education/experiences would prepare me for becoming a qualified candidate for a career like yours?
- How did you get started in this career?
- What is your schedule like on a typical day?
- Do you have on-call responsibilities? Do you travel or have overtime responsibilities/work?
- What is the potential for growth and advancement in your career?
- What skills should I be developing?
- What type of recognition do you get from your career?
- What do you like about your career? Dislike?
- To whom do you report?
- What is the salary range at the entry level? At advanced levels?
- Do you have additional recommendations of persons I may speak with about entering this career?

Screening Interview

The first interview is often a screening interview that is used by an employer to screen a number of job applicants in or out of further consideration. The screening interview is often short, 15-45 minutes, and may be conducted over the phone, by teleconference, in person, at job fairs or when you drop off a resume at the human resource office. Screening interviews by phone are on the rise. In this type interview, the interviewer cannot see your face so your voice must reflect your enthusiasm. For the teleconference interviews rehearse in advance.

It is helpful to have your resume in front of you as well as your prepared list of questions. In addition, have your portfolio ready for easy access and reference. The screening interviewer will confer with the supervisor or person with authority to hire if you are selected to move to the next step.

One-on-One Interview

The one-on-one interview is the most common interview format and is usually conducted on site by the hiring person. The interviewer focuses on questions to assess your skills, knowledge, and abilities as they relate to the career.

Search-and-Screen/Series Interview

The search and screen/series interview is rarely used for entry-level jobs. It is commonly used for more experienced positions such as management or administration. Often it usually involves a series of interviews, meeting with several individuals within the organization, one at a time or in a group situation. Following the interviews, the interviewers will compare notes and make a collective hiring decision. All the interviewers will ask questions and have equal input into the hiring decision.

Panel Interview

In a panel interview several people interview you at the same time. The panel interviewers will represent different departments and generally will ask questions that correspond to their areas of interest/expertise. Direct your answers to the person who asks the question, but maintain eye contact with the other members of the group as well. The panel interview tends to be more stressful than other types of interviews.

Peer Group Interview

This type of interview will introduce you to potential co-workers. They will evaluate you and make recommendations as to whether or not you will "fit in." However, they usually do not have the authority to hire you. Focus on being agreeable and approachable rather than someone with all the answers.

Luncheon Interview

This type of interview is to assess how well you can handle yourself in social situations. Most likely you will dine with your potential boss, co-workers, and the human resource representative. Select light, healthy, and easy things to eat. Steer clear of spaghetti in sauce and potentially messy foods that are not easy to eat gracefully. Do not order alcohol even if others do.

Videoconference Interview

This type of interview allows employers to see and judge appearance and body language to get a deeper sense of what applicants have to offer before flying them cross-country for an interview. The videoconference interview saves time and money and allows several locations to connect at once. Tips for videoconference interviews include:

- Speak up if you are experiencing any difficulty with sound, delays, or picture.
- Dress conservatively in solid colors. Keep distractions like jewelry to a minimum. Choose soft, neutral shades rather than black and white, which are too extreme on camera. Various shades of blue are good. Watch TV presenters and newscasters for other ideas about camera-ready clothes.
- Look at the camera full-face, as though you were presenting the news. Talk to the camera as you would any person interviewing you. Be conversational, maintain eye contact and smile at the camera.
- Keep your movements limited. Hand gestures will be magnified on the screen. Use small, smooth movements when gesturing.
- Focus on your purpose and presentation. You want the attention and concentration to be on you and what you are saying.
- A disadvantage of the videoconference is that there is a lag as the data is compressed and sent from one location to another. This means there is a silence while you sit and wait for a response from the other end. However you can actually watch the interviewers while answers are received. Remember not to step on the other person's words. Allow for the delay.

Second Interview

The second interview tends to be longer, involve more people, and is often held at the organization work site. A combination of individual, panel, and peer group interviews may occur during a process that may last from 1 to 2 days. The focus of the second interview is to ensure that you have the necessary skills and that you will blend well with the organization's culture.

Decision/Hiring/Placement Interview

The decision/hiring/placement interview is the kind used for making the actual hiring decision and is usually conducted by the supervisor or person with authority to hire you. It will be conducted in greater depth than the screening interview. Most applicants expect only one person to conduct the hiring/placement interview and expect it to take place in an office setting. However, it many involve several people over the course of a full day in different settings.

EMPLOYER EXPECTATIONS

Interviewers must find out certain information about the candidate and their questions are designed to elicit the information. At every point in the interview process, they are evaluating you. The following include expectations of employers.

1. Do you look like the right person?

Appearance: First impressions count!
- Personal appearance and grooming
- Manner and social skills
- Paperwork including resumes

2. Can you be counted on?

Dependability
- Comes in on time and does not abuse days off
- Can be trusted
- Gets things done on time
- Gets along well with others
- Is productive and hard working

3. Can you do the job?

Skills, Experience, Training and Education
- Has enough work experience to do the job
- Has the needed education and training
- Interests and hobbies support the job objective
- Has additional appropriate life experiences
- Shows a record of achievements
- Presents the ability to do the job

BASIC PHASES OF AN INTERVIEW

No two interviews are alike, but there are similarities. The typical interview will last 30 minutes, although some may be longer. This section will include a brief overview of what to expect and how to prepare for your successful interview. The typical structure of the interview includes:

1. Before you meet, the interviewer can form first impressions of you. You may have spoken on the phone, sent a resume or other correspondence or someone may have told the interviewer about you.

    Interview Activity: Write at least three ways that you could make a good or a bad first impression before you get to the interview.

    a. _____

    b. _____

    c. _____

2. The first few minutes of an interview are very important. If you make a bad first impression, you may not be able to change the interviewer's opinion. Usually there will be five minutes of small talk. Topics may range from your trip, weather or sports. You must talk. Being secure and confident will give you a better chance of getting the position. You are being evaluated even before the actual interview begins. See the section on communication skill in this chapter.

    Interview Activity: What do interviewers notice? List three things interviewers can observe as they first meet you that would affect their impression of you.

    a. _____

    b. _____

    c. _____

3. Fifteen minutes for you to discuss your credentials as they relate to the needs of the employer. Show that you have researched the company and emphasize that you will work as a dedicated member of the organization. Be sure you have a clear understanding of the position and the company. Listen carefully to the interviewer's questions to determine any underlying concerns and attempt to dispel them. It is important to directly address the questions asked. Emphasize your specific strengths to sell yourself as a well-balanced package. Be prepared to deal with aspects of your background that could be negative as well as positive.

Interview Activity: What are three specific ideas you have to improve your interview performance?

a. _____

b. _____

c. _____

4. Five minutes for you to ask questions. It is important to have a few questions ready when the interviewer asks if you have questions. Questions should elicit positive responses from the interviewer. Questions should bring out your interest in and knowledge of the organization. By asking well thought out questions, you show the interviewer you are serious about the organization and need more information. It also indicates that you have done your homework.

Interview Activity: List three questions that you would ask to show the interviewer(s) that you want the position.

a. _____

b. _____

c. _____

5. Five minutes to close the interview. During this time the interviewer is assessing your overall performance. Take a few minutes to summarize your key points. Remain enthusiastic and courteous. If any problems or weaknesses came up, state why they will not keep you from doing a good job. Point out the strengths you have for the position and why you believe you can do it well. Ask for the position if you are interested in it. Shake the interviewer's hand and thank the interviewer for considering you. Use the following call-back close.

Thank the interviewer by name:	While shaking hands, say "Thank you (say name) for your time today."
Express your interest:	Tell the employer that you are interested in the position, the organization, or both. An example: "The position we discussed is just what I have been looking for and I am very impressed by your organization."
Arrange a reason and a time to call back	It is important that you arrange a day and time for a follow-up call. Never expect the employer to call you. For example, say, " I'm sure I'll have questions. When would be the best time for me to get back to you?"
Say good-bye:	After you have set a date and time to call back, thank the interviewer by name and say good-bye. For example: "Thank you, Mr. (name), for the time you have spent with me today. I will call you next Wednesday morning, between 10 and 11 o'clock."

Interview Activity: Consider what you have learned about this phase of the interview and note any specific ideas to improve your interview performance.

a. _____

b. _____

c. _____

6. Follow Up. Leaving an interview does not mean it is over. By following up you can make the difference between getting the job or someone else getting it. You must:

- Send a thank-you note, no later than 24 hours after the interview. A Thank-you note (See Chapter 8) is an act of appreciation. The interviewer will most likely remember you. This indicates that you are thoughtful, well organized and thorough.

- Make notes. Write yourself notes about the interview while it is still fresh in you mind. You may not remember details a week later.

- Follow up as you promised. If you said you would call back, do it at the time designated. This will impress the interviewer on your organizational skills.

Interview Activity: Consider what you have learned in this phase of the interview and note any specific ideas to improve you interview performance.

a. _____

b. _____

c. _____

7. Negotiating Salary and Benefits. Never discuss salary until you are offered the position. Decide what you will have to have and discuss it with the interviewer. You may lose the position if you will not negotiate.

Interview Activity: The interviewer asks you, "What do you expect to get paid for this position?" What do you say? Write your response below.

a. _____

b. _____

c. _____

8. The Final Decision. The interview process is not over until you accept the position. Record the positives and the negatives about the position. Review your responses before making your final decision.

Interview Activity: Consider what you have learned about this phase of an interview and note any specific ideas to improve the decision making phase.

a. _____

b. _____

c. _____

THREE STEPS TO ANSWERING PROBLEM QUESTIONS

1. Understand what is really being asked.

- Can we depend on you?
- Are you easy to get along with?
- Are you a good worker?
- Do you have the experience and training to do the job if we hire you?

2. Answer the question briefly and in a non-damaging way.

- Acknowledge the facts.
- But present them as advantages, not disadvantages.

3. Answer the real concern by presenting your knowledge and skills.

- Base your answer on your key skills and abilities.
- Give examples to support your statements.

TOP TWELVE INTERVIEW QUESTIONS

The interviewer will observe and evaluate you during the entire interview process. S/he wants to find out if you are mentally alert, have intellectual depth when communicating, have the capacity for problem-solving, and how well you respond to stress and pressure? When you respond to questions or ask your own questions, your statements should be concise and organized without being too brief. Let's review some tips for answering the top most frequently asked interview questions.

1. Can you tell me a little about yourself?

This is an open-ended question usually asked to help "break the ice." Remember to keep your response short and related to the position. Your answer should be about 2 minutes in length. The interviewer wants you to tell how your background relates to doing the job. Give a brief personal history and then get right into your relevant skills and experiences. Examples of responses include:

Example # 1: With Work Experience

My name is _____. I am pursuing a bachelor's degree in _____ at _____University. My courses have enabled me to gain essential knowledge in (list specific areas of your major). I have utilized this knowledge as a (job title/project) where I (brief description of duties). I have additional work experience. I also have _____ years of experience as a(n) _____ where I have enhanced my knowledge and skills in (list subject areas). My employment interests include (list professions of interest).

Example # 2: Without Work Experience

My name is _____. I am pursuing a bachelor's degree in (major) at _____ University. My courses have enabled me to gain essential knowledge in (list specific areas of your major). Throughout my studies I have (list any honors, campus/community activities and memberships). (Example: Throughout my studies I have maintained a 3.0 grade point average, been inducted into the Beta Kappa Chi National Honor Society and served a term as Student Government Association Vice-President.). These activities have helped me _____ (Example: These activities and involvement have helped me to build my communication skills and taught me the importance of teamwork.). My employment interests include (list professions of interest).

Interview Activity: Use the three basic step process to answer this question.

a. _____

b. _____

c. _____

2. Why should I hire you?

Why should anyone hire you? Maybe this question is not asked this frankly but this is the question behind many interview questions. The best answer is to show the employer that you have done your homework. Be specific and state how what you have learned about the school/organization through your research relates to your career goals. Show you can solve a problem for them, help the school/organization or provide something else of value that they need. Think about the most valuable thing you can do for an organization/school.

3. What are your major strengths/weakness?

Describe strengths that are in some way related to the position you are applying for or your work style in general. Always present any perceived weakness in a positive manner. For instance, " I tend to have a difficult time saying "no", and when I get too much on my plate, I can get a little stressed. Recently, I've asked my friend to help me monitor this and it's working out fine. I'm proud to say; I have been able to say "no" a lot lately." Another example is, "I tend to be nervous around my principal, and although I've gained more confidence in that area since my last job where my principal encouraged me to ask questions." Again make yourself sound good.

4. How would you describe your best/worst boss?

Be careful and be positive. Respond in a way that indicates your respect for authority and your ability to get along with superiors. Speak about your best boss with little emphasis on your worst boss. If pressed to speak about your worst boss, try to put a positive spin on it. For instance, "I had a principal who was often very vague. However, because of this, I learned the value of good communication skills."

5. What are your plans for the future?

Tell the interviewer that you hope to be with the school/organization in whatever capacity you can make the greatest contribution based on the skills and experience you have gained over the course of the preceding years. Employers are concerned about investing time and money into employees who will leave the organization after a short time on the job. Place yourself in the employer's position and then answer the questions.

6. What is an example of a problem you encountered in school or at work? Explain how you solved it.

Be logical. State the problem and then illustrate the step-by-step procedure you used to correct it.

7. What is the name of the last book you read?

The interviewer intends to see if you remain current in your field and/or read for self-improvement. Think of (and read) a book that relates to your career or contributes to your personal growth.

8. What sort of pay do you expect to receive?

Research what others in the school/organization make. Contact professional organizations and get their annual salary surveys. Read professional publications. Network and look on the Web to find out what others in your career are making. Every employer has some type of salary range in mind. Find out the range before you state any salary requirements. Consider the following points when negotiating salary:

Rule 1: Never discuss salary until you are being offered the job. Suppose the employer was willing to pay you $20,000 per year and you say you will take $18,000, guess what you will be paid? You may get screened out early in the interview by discussing salary too soon.

Rule 2: Know the probably salary range in advance. Before the interview, you need to know what similar jobs in similar types of organizations pay. This will give you an idea of what the position is likely to pay. Ask others in similar jobs. Ask the research librarian in the library for salary information. Also contact your local state Employment Service's statistical office. They are required to keep this information for each area.

Rule 3: Bracket your salary range. Your research finds that the employer pays between $18,000 and $24,000 per year, state your own range as "high teens to mid-twenties." This covers the amount the employer probably had in mind and gives you room to get more. The following examples apply for any salary range, so simply translate the concept and apply it to the salary range that makes sense for you.

Table 7.1   Examples of Salary Range

Examples of Salary Range	
If They Pay:	**You Say:**
$7/hour	6 to 8 dollars per hour
$15,000/year	mid-to upper teens
$18,000/year	upper teens to low twenties
$22,000/year	low to mid-twenties
$27,500/year	upper twenties to low thirties
$90,000/year	high five figure to low six figure

Rule 4: Never say no to a job immediately after the offer is made. Wait until at least 24 hours have passed. Remember the objective of an interview is to get a job offer.

9.   What will your former employers (or references) say about you?

The interviewer wants to know about your adaptive skills and whether you can be depended on. Are you easy to get along with? Are you reliable? Many employers will check your references. The interviewer will likely find out any of your past problems, so be honest.

10. Probing Questions Interviewer May Ask

Often times many of the questions that are asked in the interview are designed to uncover your underlying qualities. The interviewer may not ask a question that directly addresses the information s/he is looking for, but may gather it from your response. Examples of these type questions are listed below and in Table 7.2.

Table 7.2   Probing Questions

Questions Establishing Honest/Integrity
• Discuss a time when your integrity was challenged. How did you handle it? • What would you do if someone asked you to do something unethical? • In what business situations do you feel honesty would be inappropriate? • If you saw a co-worker doing something dishonest, what would you do? • How do you measure your own success?
Questions Revealing Personality/Ability to Work With Others
• Do you consider yourself a risk taker? • What kind of environment would you like to work in? • What kinds of responsibilities would you like to avoid in your next job? • What are two or three examples of tasks that you do not particularly enjoy doing? Indicate how you remain motivated to complete those tasks. • Tell me about a work situation that irritated you. • Have you ever had a conflict with a co-worker? How did you resolve it? • How do you think your subordinates perceive you? • What previous job was the most satisfying and why? • What job was the most frustrating and why?
Questions Revealing Past Mistakes and Ownership of Mistakes
• Tell me about an objective in your last job that you failed to meet and why? • What have you learned from your mistakes? • Tell me about a situation where you abruptly had to change what you were doing. • Tell me of a time when you had to work on a project that didn't work out as expected? What did you do? • If you had the opportunity to change anything in your career, what would you have done differently?
Questions Revealing Problem Solving
• What have you done that was innovative? • What was the wildest idea you had in the past year? What did you do about it? • Describe a situation in which you had a difficult problem. How did you solve it? • Describe some situations in which you worked under pressure or met deadlines. • When taking on a new task, do you like to have a great deal of feedback and responsibility at the outset or do you like to try your own approach?

11. Sample Responses To Personal Questions

The following are some sample responses to direct or indirect questions about your personal situation. The responses that follow are all simple, direct, and positive. Each one also allows you to quickly move to presenting your skills.

Young children at home
"I have two children, both in school. Child care is no problem since they stay with a good friend."

Single head of household
"I'm not married and have two children at home. It is very important to me to have a steady income, and child care is no problem."

Young and single
"I'm not married, and if I should marry, that would not change my plans for a full-time career. For now, I can devote my full attention to my career."

Just moved here
"I've decided to settle here in (location) permanently. I've rented an apartment, and the moving vans are unloading there now."

Relatives, childhood
"I had a good childhood. Both of my parents still live within an hour's flight from here, and I see them several times a year."

Leisure
"For relaxation I grow a garden in my spare time and am a member of the Garden Club organization."
My time is family-centered when I'm not working. I'm also active in several community organizations and spend at least some time each week in church activities."

12. Why are you looking for this sort of position and why here?

This question provides you with the opportunity to show how well you researched the position or organization. Indicate what specifically about your research caused you to be interested in working for this organization or company. This is a chance for you to show how your career goals are related to working for them.

SEVEN STEPS TO EFFECTIVE PREPARATION

Your approach the job interview is the single most important step to getting the job. The seven steps which will help you be well prepared for the interview include:

1. **Research the employer, position, field and interview situation.** Research the employer thoroughly. Read current periodicals and professional journals to learn about current trends in the field. Read company literature, mission statements, and annual reports. Be familiar with the employer's organizational structure. Write down important facts and study these facts. Become very familiar with the gathered information. Prepare for the interview situation by getting information such as:

   - Name, title, telephone number, business address of the trip coordinator
   - Directions and correct address of the interview site
   - Itinerary for the day
   - Details of the travel arrangements: hotel, airline ticket, auto rental, area map, etc.
   - Name of person responsible for making travel arrangements
   - Financial arrangements for trip (Will organization pay? Will you pay? Will you be reimbursed?)
   - Exact time and location of interview
   - Name of individual you should report to upon your arrival
   - Names and titles of individuals who will interview you
   - Interview format/agenda?

2. **Match your strengths to the organizations profile.** Relate the strength of the organization to your own strengths and professional needs. Think about your skills, interests, and values and consider your strengths and weaknesses. Be able to discuss decisions you have made and the thought behind them. Be able to identify accomplishments you are proud of and things you might have done differently. At the interview, you will need to convey your message of how you will add to this organizational team by demonstrating knowledge and understanding of its philosophy and goals.

3. **Prepare a list of key questions to ask the interviewer.** Learn about the interviewing organization. It is acceptable to bring a written list of questions to the interview to use as a reference. The visit/tour is your chance to learn and gather information from the organization itself, your chance to interview them. This kind of preparation is likely to impress rather than to indicate a weakness. Some commonly asked questions by the interviewer include:

   - What do employees like best about the organization? Least?
   - How much employee turnover is there?
   - What are the living conditions in this area of the country?
   - How large is the department in which the opening exists? How is it organized?
   - Why is the position open?
   - How much travel would normally be expected?
   - What type of training program/orientation does a new employee receive? Who conducts it? When does it start and end?
   - What are the long-range possibilities for employees in similar positions who consistently perform above expectations?
   - What are the major responsibilities of the department? Of the job?
   - What would the new employee be expected to have accomplished in the first six months on the job? The first year?
   - What are the special projects now ongoing in the department? What are some that are coming in the future?
   - Describe the chain of command. To whom would I report?
   - What goes on during a typical workday?
   - How much interaction is there with superiors? Colleagues? Clients? How much independent work is there?
   - Do you have a formal training program? If so, please describe your training process.
   - What characteristics are you looking for in the person to fill this position?
   - Would you describe your company's management philosophy?
   - What do you consider to be the major problem facing your organization at this time?
   - How often are performance reviews given?
   - Where have the last three people who held this position gone?

4. **Be prepared.** The more thorough your research, the better idea you have of the type of questions you will be asked in the interview. Attend an interviewing skills workshop and read books on interviewing skills. Often times a tough interviewer will ask a question designed to test your reaction to a negative comment. Think about the question before you answer. Slang, street talk, and, of course, profanity, should be avoided at all costs. Don't embellish, brag or provide more information than is requested. And don't rush your answers. Eye contact is part of your demeanor that can either count for or against you. Answer questions thoughtfully; don't just react to the questions. Some questions an interviewer may ask are:

   - **Personal Questions**
     - What can you tell me about yourself?
     - Why did you choose to interview with our organization? What do you know about us?
     - What can you offer us?
     - If I spoke to your former employer, what would he/she say would be your greatest strengths? Weaknesses?
     - Of which three accomplishments are you most proud? Who are your role models? Why?
     - What motivates you most in a job?
     - Why should we hire you?
     - Where do you want to be in five years? Ten?
     - How did your college education or work experience prepare you for this position?

- **Education Related Questions**
  - Why did you choose to attend your college/university?
  - Why did you choose this major?
  - Do your grades reflect you ability? Why? Why not?
  - Which classes in your major did you like best? Least? Why?
  - What were some of the campus activities in which you participated?
  - Did you financially assist yourself during your college/university education?

- **Career Goals**
  - What kind of supervisor do you prefer?
  - Do you prefer large or small organizations? Why?
  - Are you able to work on several assignments at one time?
  - Do you have any problems about working overtime?
  - Do you have problems with traveling?
  - How do you feel about relocating?
  - Are you willing to work flextime?
  - Do you prefer to work on your own or under supervision?

5. **Practice for the interview.** Before beginning the interview, practice answering questions. Tape your answers, either on audio or video, and review your "practice interview." Pay attention to what you said and also to how you said it. Tape yourself again to see if you have improved. Ask a friend, instructor or career advisor to interview you in a "mock interview" situation. Ask that person to critique your performance, how you answer the questions, what kind of an impression you make, how you present yourself through your body language, voice tone, eye contact, and general demeanor. Also, attend an interviewing workshop and meet with a counselor to review your interview strategy. Participate in a "Freeze Frame," a video taped mock interview and review interview questions with a friend or faculty member.

6. **Learn proper interview conduct.** Be prepared to conduct yourself in a professional manner during the interview. The way you sit, hold your head, fold your arms, cross your legs and what you do with your hands, affects your interview style. For example:

- Answering a question in the positive way, while shaking your head "no" (a very common habit) sends a mixed message to the listener.
- A woman in a skirt, sitting across from the interviewer, needs to be in a modest position, so as to relieve any potential distraction.
- Folding your arms across your chest is a subtle way of "shutting out" the person to whom you are talking.

The following is a list of some of the factors you should keep in mind in the interview process:

- Plan to arrive for the interview at least ten minutes before the scheduled start time but no more than fifteen minutes early. Arriving early will allow you to step into the restroom and check yourself in a full-length mirror to ensure that hair and clothes are properly in place. Ladies it is smart to carry an extra pair of hose in your purse. Tidying up a bit can boost your confidence and preclude needless embarrassment. This may be an opportune time to use a breath freshener.
- The dress guidelines for on-campus interviews apply also to office/organization interviews. Refer to Dress for Success later in this chapter.
- If you smoke, don't smoke while at the organization or in the presence of organization employees.
- The employer begins to evaluate you the minute you are identified. When you meet the employer, give a good, firm handshake and be sure to make eye contact as you exchange introductions and greetings. Don't be afraid to extend your hand first. This shows assertiveness.
- Ordering alcoholic beverages at a business lunch or dinner is an issue to avoid. As a general rule, unless you are interviewing with an organization that has a stake in such beverages, it is better to ask for something other than alcohol.
- Brush up on your table manners. Organizations look for social skills as well as those needed for the job, especially if the job entails close contacts with the organization's clients.

- During "small talk" with interviewers, try to avoid controversial topics like politics and religion. Your stated position may help or hurt your chances for a job offer.
- Carry several copies of your resume to give to others who may interview you. Bring a separate, typed list of at least three references, each with the name, title, address, fax number, e-mail and phone number, plus the most suitable time each can be reached. References used should have an academic or professional relationship with you, not just a personal one.
- Bring with you any supporting material you may have, such as letters of recommendation, certifications, transcripts, or published papers or projects. Some supervisors prefer to look at transcripts at the time of the interview, if not before.
- Take mental notes as you go through the interview. At the end of the interview make a short concise summary of your qualifications and stress your interest in the position. Thank the interviewer for taking the time to meet with you and ask if you could call in a few days to check on the status of your application.

7. **Look back when the interview is over.** The interviewing process is not finished when the interview is over. Immediately following the interview, go over the questions you had. Rethink how you could answer them better if they're ever asked again. Practice your revised answers aloud. Write down as many details about the interview as you can remember.

Thank you letters are the final step in the interviewing process and most employers are impressed by this professional courtesy. Type a thank-you letter within two or three days to the interviewer and to any others who may have spent time answering your questions. A thank-you note once again places your name in front of the interviewer and reemphasizes your interest in the job and your major attributes. A thank you letter should be short and reaffirms your interest in the position and the organization; it also is a time to sell your qualifications one more time.

If you receive no word from the organization in a week or so after your thank-you, call to check the status of the employee search. Call the person who interviewed you and ask if you can answer any further questions or send any additional material. If you are invited for a second interview, know that you have a 50-50 chance of receiving a job offer. Prepare a list on specific issues rather than on the general one you talked about previously. The subjects of salary, benefits, bonuses, and options will be open for discussion, but probably not until after an offer has been extended.

Seldom will you get an offer while at the organization but it does happen. Don't say "yes" until you have had the time to think about it, even though you want the position and do plan to accept it. Be gracious in your thanks for the offer, but ask for some time to consider it. Do you have other applications in the works? You do not want to miss a better offer that might come from one of the other organizations. Give it a few days until you can give the organization an unqualified "yes" or "no" in deference to another organization's better offer.

DECLINING AN OFFER

Whether the compensation is too low, the location is not where you wish to live or the job is not the right one sometime you just need to say, "Thanks, but no thanks." Life is too short to make decisions that are going to make you miserable. The best way to handle difficult decisions is to weigh the consequences and decide what is best for you. It is tempting to verbally turn down an offer and not write a letter but it is more professional to write a formal letter to decline the offer. Refer to Chapter 8 for an example of a declining an offer letter (Withdrawal Letter). Keep these tips in mind as you write your letter.

- Be prompt. As soon as you make your decision, call the hiring person and write your letter declining the offer.
- The employer needs to offer the position to someone else and you don't want to hold up the process. Be courteous.
- You may turn this position down but in the future you might want to be considered for other opportunities.
- Thank each person with whom you interviewed and wish them and their company continued success. This is good networking for future opportunities.
- Be diplomatic. Convey to the hiring person that you were impressed by the school/organization and you carefully considered the offer, but you are accepting a position that better suits your career objectives.
- Be concise. Keep your letter short and sweet. The company already realizes your value since they wanted to hire you.

INTERVIEWING AFTER A JOB LOSS

Maybe you were laid off, fired or you had differences in opinion with your employer and coworkers. Now you are looking to your first post-layoff interview. A positive, forward-looking attitude impresses employers, thus a negative attitude can be a turnoff. Prepare by researching the school/organization and position for which you are interviewing. Being prepared shows that you are professional, mature and worthy of being considered. Unprepared candidates give the appearance of being disorganized and unprofessional and only reinforce any impression a bad reference might give. Remember the dos in a job search.

Dos

- Do contact former employers who thought well of you and who will give you a good reference to obtain letters of recommendation.

- Do prepare for hard questions and practice answers you would give if asked. Have relatives and friends listen to your answers and give their opinion on how the answers sound.

- Do know your accomplishments and value. Believe that you do bring value and skills to prospective employers.

- Do spend time thinking about what you accomplished and skills you bring to the table. Make a list and review it several times. This will help improve your self-confidence and your attitude at your interview.

- Do discuss your accomplishments instead of the negative aspects of your previous job. Discuss what you learned from the experience that will make you a better employee in the future.

- Do keep searching and don't get discouraged. The reason you did not get a job may have nothing to do with you.

- Write to the interviewer to find out why you were not hired. Make it clear you are not trying to change the decision but are trying to get information that will help you in your job search. Learn from each interview and continue searching.

COMMUNICATION SKILLS

Communication is a key element in all interviews. It is up to you to modify your communication style so the interviewer will be comfortable and receptive to you.

Verbal Skills

What you say and how you say it conveys the messages that you are giving during the interview.

- Listen carefully to what is being asked and answer the question.
- Use clear, concise answers.
- Use proper grammar. Avoid use of slang or colloquialisms.
- Be positive.
- Be specific; refer to concrete experiences
- Avoid salary and benefit issues unless the employer brings up the subject.

Nonverbal Skills

Nonverbal skills give a clear message. Be aware of the message that you are giving with your body language and facial expressions. Positive nonverbal communication factors will reinforce your verbal message.

- Give a firm handshake to the interviewer.
- Maintain steady eye contact with the interviewer.
- Use positive facial expressions and vocal qualities.
- Sit attentively to demonstrate your interest and enthusiasm. If you have a choice, sit in the chair furthest away from the door. This indicates that you are comfortable and self-confident.
- Dress in a professional manner to convey a polished, professional image.

Listening Skills

Calvin Coolidge once said, "No man ever listened himself out of a job." To be more successful, you must be a better listener. Hourly employees may spend 30 percent of their time listening, while managers often spend 60 percent, and executives 75 percent or more.   Speakers share their wisdom and try to persuade, while listeners make meaning of what is heard—they make the ultimate decision to act on what they hear.

- **A Good Listener:**

  - Uses eye contact appropriately
  - Is attentive and alert to a speaker's verbal and nonverbal behavior
  - Is patient and doesn't interrupt (waits for speaker to finish)
  - Is responsive, using verbal and nonverbal expressions
  - Asks questions in a non-threatening tone
  - Paraphrases, restates or summarizes what the speaker says
  - Provides constructive (verbal or nonverbal) feedback
  - Is empathic (works to understand the speaker)
  - Shows interest in the speaker as a person
  - Demonstrates a caring attitude and is willing to listen
  - Doesn't criticize, is nonjudgmental
  - Is open-minded

- **A Poor Listener:**

  - Interrupts the speaker (is impatient)
  - Doesn't give eye contact (eyes wander)
  - Is distracted (fidgeting) and does not pay attention to the speaker
  - Is not interested in the speaker (daydreaming)
  - Gives the speaker little or no feedback (verbal or nonverbal)
  - Changes the subject
  - Is judgmental
  - Is closed-minded
  - Talks too much
  - Is self-preoccupied.
  - Gives unwanted advice
  - Is too busy to listen

ILLEGAL QUESTIONS

Federal, state, and local laws regulate the types of questions a prospective employer may ask. Questions asked during the interview and listed on the job application must be related to the job for which you are applying. Questions should address only what the employer needs to know to decide whether or not you can perform the functions of the job. Refer to Chapter 9 Legal Issues for information concerning illegal questions.

10 TIPS FOR A POSITIVE INTERVIEW

1. Use the interviewer's name - title and last name - from time to time as you speak. Avoid using the interviewer's first name unless you have been requested to do so.
2. Phrase your questions so that you sound sure of yourself. "What would be my duties?" sounds more assertive than "What are the duties of the job?"
3. Use good grammar and good diction. Say "yes," not "yeah."
4. Listen to how quickly you speak and look for moderation. Avoid talking too fast or too slowly.
5. Avoid filling pauses with "um," "Uh," or "ah," don't punctuate sentences with "you know," "like," "see," or "okay."
6. Punctuate your speech just as you would a sentence. Stress the words that are most important. Don't arbitrarily emphasize every third word. Project your voice loudly enough to be heard. Watch the tone of your voice. Articulate clearly, do not mumble.
7. Use active words.
8. Avoid using words that sound indecisive such as: "think," "guess," or "feel." Also, avoid "pretty good" or "fairly well." Talk about yourself and your skills with positive words.
9. Offer examples of your accomplishments. Use illustrations, descriptions, statistics, and testimonials to support your claims
10. Keep your shoulders back, head erect, and avoid folding your arms across your chest, and sitting or standing with arms or legs far apart or what could be described as an open position. Sit with a very slight forward lean toward the interviewer, make eye contact frequently, but don't overdo it. A moderate amount of smiling will help reinforce your positive image. Listen well. Listening is a learned skill. Being a good listener takes effort.

EVALUATING A JOB OFFER

You have received the news that you were selected for the position and all the hours you spent job searching and interviewing have paid off. Before you telephone the personnel department, wait. Make certain that you think about it before making this major decision in your life.

Guidelines to evaluate your job offer include:

- Always ask for time to think it over. Review the offer with a friend or family and ask for suggestions about negotiating a better financial package.
- Before you begin the negotiation process research the marketplace and salary range for a person with your background and experience. The best resource for information on salary is the Career Development Center on your campus.
- Carefully consider your finances: how much you would like to earn, need to earn, the opportunity the position presents and the potential for raises and career progression within the school system. Be realistic about what the school system can offer and how that fits your needs. There are non-cash items and, if you will be moving to a different city, relocation issues to consider also. Figure 6.6 lists some of the non-cash items to consider.

Figure 7.6   Non-cash items

HEALTH AND LIFE INSURANCE PROGRAMS	RETIREMENT AND EMPLOYEE ASSISTANCE
Family Life Insurance Family Health Insurance Dismemberment Insurance Accidental Death	Retirement Benefits, Financial Problems Employee Counseling Family Counseling Substance abuse
VACATIONS	EDUCATIONAL PROGRAMS
Supplemental Vacation Personal Leave, number of days the first year Paid Holidays Compensation for Unused Days Carry-over or Accrual Provisions	Tuition Reimbursement Education/Training Expenses Professional Association Membership Subscriptions to Professional Journals

Relocation Factors

A new job is a learning opportunity and so is living in a different section of the country. Relocation will be a part of many of our careers. You should learn to think nationally as well as internationally. In our mobile society, it is common for people to move from one state to another, not only to new job opportunities but also to completely new careers. You should weigh the factors listed in Figure 7.7 before you make this important change in your life.

Seal the Deal

After you have given in depth thought to the offer, it is time to seal the deal. Agree on a decision date and be sure to give your answer by that date. If possible, try to get the employer to "put it in writing." Be certain that no "contingencies" remain up in the air. For example, have all reference and security checks been made? Sound your trumpet about your new job... only when you are "on board." Once you have started your job, call or write the people with whom you negotiated to thank them for their time and interest. Thank the many people who helped you during your job search. You may need them again.

Figure 7.7   Relocation Factors

RELOCATION FACTORS	
Salary	Comparative cost of living
Relocation expenses	Transportation
Religious opportunities	Environmental quality
Spouse/family concerns	Social/cultural activities
Climate	Political climate
Availability/quality of schools	Population size
Availability/cost of homes	

DRESS FOR SUCCESS

"Clothes make the man." In today's politically correct society, it would be more appropriate to say, "Clothes make the person." In other words, how a person dresses makes a statement about one's self-identification, image conveyed to others, and level of occupational aspiration. In fact, for those who strive to obtain the best careers following graduation and achieve progression later on are advised to dress for success.

John Molloy, author and lecturer of seminars for "Dress For Success," states that years and years of research have proven that one's chances for success in any given business and social situation is affected by the clothes s/he wears, the body language that s/he exhibits, as well as her/his knowledge of the situation. Most important decisions are made about people of all ethnicities, ages, and abilities based on their appearance and demeanor when s/he interviews for a job.

First impressions can be very difficult to change. In the first ten seconds of meeting a candidate, the interviewer makes a mental decision on whether you look right for the job. Make the best first impression. First impressions are lasting. You have one change to make a good impression, don't blow it! At the moment that you step inside the place of employment, all eyes will be focused on you, including the receptionist. These people will draw some opinion of you based on how you dress, present yourself and fit in with the group based on your grooming, attire, and personal department. Dressing for the workplace is not a fashion show; however, you want to display tasteful quality in your dress style. Clothes reflect your confidence, capability, competence, and credibility, as well as your best physical attributes. The way you look and the way you present yourself has a lot to do with whether or not the employer is comfortable with trusting you, feeling you are competent, or is okay with the idea of you meeting his or her customers. Your professional appearance and your verbal skills are most important. An attaché or leather briefcase will enhance your professional look.

Appropriate Dress for Men

Two-piece single-breasted suits, solid colors (navy blue and gray); and tighter-woven fabrics are safer than bold prints or patterns. Bright ties bring focus to the face, but a simple pattern is best for an interview. How well your clothes look is a major factor of your appearance. The proper fit is smooth, so the clothes do not wrinkle easily or look tight or baggy. A tailor or a clothing department alternations department can make your clothes fit properly.

- Well-pressed, two-piece dark suit (navy or charcoal) made with nice fabric such as blended wool. A college stripe is the most universally acceptable style.
- Bottom edge of slacks should just touch the top of the shoes in the front, then angle to three-quarters of an inch (3/4") longer in the back.
- Long-sleeved, white cotton shirt with tab, button-down, spread, or standard point collar (polyester blends are out). White goes well with any color combinations and is a must for formal occasions. Solid color of light blue, tan, cream, and light gray are good choices. For striped shirts, choose blue, tan and gray.
- Use the suit color as the base color, and the shirt and tie as the accent color. Match the shirts to one of the colors in a tie.
- Colorful silk tie that is not too flashy (red) . Ties should fall no lower than top of the belt buckle. For solid color or patterned suits, choose solid colored shirts and solid colored or patterned ties. The best looking neckties are wool, polyester blend but preferably silk. A properly tied necktie should be symmetrically knotted.
- Black socks high enough so the skin is not visible when you sit down and cross your legs.
- Well-shined black shoes (lace-up wing tip or box toe is preferred). Never wear brown shoes or loafers to an interview.
- Matching leather black or brown belt

Appropriate Dress for Women

Women have many more alternatives in their professional wardrobes, from a simple cut dress, to a skirt and blouse or a tailored dress with or without a jacket, to suits. Select clothing of classic designs, which is conservative in appearance and made of quality fabrics that hold their shape.

Soft, feminine skirts and blouses, sweater and skirt combinations are suggested fashion for women in the workplace. Suits with knee-length skirt and a tailored blouse are most appropriate. Pants are more acceptable now but are not recommended for interviews or unless you are positive that they would be appropriate. Avoid low-cut blouses, mini-skirts, or tight fitting clothing because this type of attire projects a non-professional appearance and weakens your credibility.

- A traditional (plain) dark two-piece business suit with medium-length skirt, not pants, are always a safe bet, but wearing a conservative business dress with tasteful accessories can also serve the purpose.
- Dark solids are more appropriate than pastels or prints.
- Light-colored blouse, neutral-colored hose.
- Style, material, color and proper fit are important in selecting shoes. Dark (preferably black) mid-heel shoes (leather shoes are most durable). Shoe style should be conservative and versatile. Sneakers, moccasins, and sandals are unacceptable.
- Handbag and shoes should match or coordinate whenever possible.
- Accent the basic attire with a colorful belt or scarf.

How do you know which way to dress? Research through library resources and Internet is an excellent way to find up-to-date information about proper dress. Also, find someone who works in the situation and ask them about the culture and how things are done. It is acceptable to call the Personnel Department and tell them that you are considering applying for employment and ask them about acceptable attire.

Hair, Teeth and Fingernails

A hair cut, a shave, a manicure, a light touch with the makeup, a good brushing and some mouthwash is basic. The interviewer will definitely notice the fingernails. They should be neat, clean and of an appropriate length. For women, a light-colored nail polish adds a nice touch. Often times it's this kind of personal hygiene that costs people a chance at a job they really prefer.

Tattoos and Body Piercings

Popular culture has made these fashionable in the social and casual settings. In corporate America, it is best to cover your tattoos and piercings with long-sleeved shirts, blouses, collars, etc. Avoid nose, eyebrow, and lip rings or anything that diverts attention from you as a professional. Any aspect of your personal image that sparks controversy can cost you the job. Be on the safe side, blend in with the more conservative elements of the company.

Ethnocentric Look

Many ethnic groups face a quandary when deciding how ethnocentric their personal wardrobe and image should be in the workplace. Many organizations respect ethnocentric individuality and accept this standard of professional attire. However, be aware of what is acceptable.

Casual Dress

Relaxed workplace attire is becoming the norm and many companies are having "Casual Friday" not only on Friday's but also for the rest of the week. Men should avoid attire such as shorts, sandals, t-shirts with words or pictures, athletic wear, worn-out jeans, and dress shirts worn as casual shirts. Women should avoid ultra-baggy pants or too small t-shirts or sweaters, leggings in place of pants or skirts, casual shorts (tailored shorts may be acceptable), open-toed sandals and gym shoes.

Accessories

Travel light and carry only one item: either a briefcase, laptop, or a leather notebook. A briefcase or laptop is recommended because it adds to the candidate's stature. A briefcase or laptop is a symbol that indicates that the individual has done some research and is probably going to be able to give the employer whatever is needed. In fact, a briefcase or laptop shows that the candidate is prepared. Use a high quality leather grain (no vinyl) attaché' case when carrying your portfolio.

For men, to be on the safe side, regardless of location or industry, take off the earring until you are well established on the job and determine that it's acceptable to express you self-identification in that way. Do not carry a small masculine clutch, save it until after you get the job

Women's accessories should be minimal. Wearing multiple rings, bracelets and earrings don't convey a conservative image. Simple gold or silver jewelry, such as a lapel pin, a watch, simple styled earrings, or a slender chain necklace with or without a pendant is acceptable. Avoid costume or faddish jewelry because of its negative impact. As a rule of thumb, two items of complementary jewelry should suffice as appropriate accessories for any interview attire. Choose a conservative style and size purse, which should be made of good quality leather. It is important to never leave your handbag on a desk, conference table (during a meeting) or on a table (during a meal). It should be stowed away, out of sight.

Dress Codes

In Corporate America, each organization has its own dress code that can range from casual (jobs in arts, scientist, etc.) to conservative (banks, law firm, etc.). Some regions of the U.S. are more formal than others, i.e., more formal in New York and Atlanta than in California and Florida. Your best choice is to find out if there is a dress code before you go to a particular organization (contact personnel department). If you interview at the organization, observe what the professional employees wear or ask the interviewer what is considered appropriate attire. Showing that you are serious about making a good impression is a very positive point to make in the interview as well as on the job.

Dressing for success means more than buying a few suits for interviewing purposes. Build a career wardrobe, carefully select clothing and accessories that mix and match well and that convey a sense of confidence, self-assurance and individuality. In clothing selection, quality always trumps quantity.

 If you need help with coordinating your wardrobe, consider consulting fashion publications, on-staff department or specialty store fashion consultants, friends or relatives who have obvious fashion sense.

Dressing For The New Job

Now you have the job. What to wear will be the first of many important decisions you will make each day. It is time for you to learn how to succeed at this job. The world of work is filled with unwritten rules of how to dress for your organization. It is the first impression that people will have when they interact with you face to face and it is the image they will keep in their minds when they have later contact on the phone or through mail or e-mail.
When you dress in the business attire it means that you have a better chance of being thought of as serious-minded.
Tips that can help you dress for your new job include:

• Schedule haircuts at regular intervals. Your hair is one accessory that you take with you every day, everywhere. Pay a little extra for a quality haircut.

• Press your clothing. Even permanent press clothes need that "finished" look.

• Keep a "business professional" outfit at the office for emergencies. Suppose it is your company's "casual" day, and a client request a last-minute meeting. Rather than attend the meeting in the wrong attire, keep a business professional outfit ready.

- **Men and Women**

  - Maintain a consistent hair color. Constantly changing it confuses people.
  - Keep your jacket on in an office environment when addressing outside clients or your supervisor/boss.
  - If you lose or gain weight have your clothes altered to keep the fit.
  - Avoid wearing too much fragrance. Many people are allergic or sensitive to overdone scents. It's better to skip cologne.
  - Avoid wearing too much jewelry that can be distracting if bulky or oversized.

- **Men**

  - Button your American-cut blazer or jacket when you stand to give that polished look. Wear a long-sleeved shirt with your jacket.
  - Wear socks that cover your calves.
  - Wear an undershirt under your dress shirt. An undershirt makes a white shirt look whiter, adds body to the dress shirt, keeps even a lightly starched shirt from itching and it protects the dress shirt from perspiration.
  - Wear a long-sleeved shirt with your jacket.

- **Women**

  - Avoid wearing more than 13 accessories. Earrings (one per ear), necklace and rings (one per hand on your ring or pinky fingers, unless you are wearing an engagement ring and wedding band), watch on one wrist and bracelet on another, your belt, and any ornate buttons on your outfit.
  - Avoid wearing skirts that are shorter in length on business casual days than you do on business professional days. Look like you mean business so you can grow within your organization is important.
  - Avoid wearing slacks to work if you have never seen top-level women at your organization wear them
  - Avoid wearing hosiery and shoes that are darker than your hem. Choose hosiery and shoes that either match the color of your hemline or are lighter. Wear skin-toned hosiery when your business outfit consists of a short-sleeved jacket or dress. This will give you a balanced look by having as much of your legs showing as your arms.

Men and women, your real taste in clothes comes out on "business casual days." Your business casual wardrobe should consist of the same type of clothes and accessories described in your organization's business casual dress code policy. If your organization does not have a documented business casual code, emulate the dress of the person whose position you want.

- Wear shoes that are well maintained. The way you take care of your shoes indicates if you pay attention to detail or have a tendency to let things go.

- Dress for the position you want, not the position you have. You must look the part to assume a position.

SUMMARY

The interview is a test to evaluate a person's professionalism and their seriousness about a job. The interviewing process may at times be an over-whelming experience for the entry level as well as the experienced professional. To get a job offer, you will need to be a dedicated, well prepared, well educated professional, and loyal. Do your preparation on the organization for the open position to be certain of all the details about the visit. Remember the basics of what you need to know about your employer as well as letting the interviewers discover what they need to know about you. In short, you should be yourself, but by all means fit in where you want to launch your career as a budding professional. If you can do all of this with professionalism and confidence, you are sure to become a top candidate for the job. Presenting the best possible image of you is imperative to gain interview success.

REFLECTIONS

1. In small groups, discuss and list the types of questions that you might expect when interviewing for a teaching position. Hold mock interviews. Use Laboratory 7.1 for your response.

2. Explore a variety of on-line sites related to the job interview. Generate a list of ten (10) sites not listed in the Web Feature section of the chapter. Use Laboratory 7.2 for your response.

WEB SITES

www.asktheinterviewcoach.com
Job Interview Questions

www.jobweb.com
Secrets to Interview Success
Interview checklist
Interviewing types and tips
Interview Q & A
Starting Salary expectations

http://editorial.careers.msn.com/articles/interview/
MSN Careers – Interviewing After a Job Loss

http://editorial.careers.msn.com/articles/video/
MSN Careers – Smile, You're on Camera: videoconference Interviews
http://editorial.careers.msn.com/articles/ask/
MSN Careers – Do You Have Any Questions?

http://editorial.careers.msn.com/articles/declining/
MSN Careers- Thanks, But No Thanks: Turning Down the Offer

http://editorial.careers.msn.com/articles/declining/
MSN Careers – Declining an Offer

http://editorial.careers.msn.com/articles/interviewquestions/
MSN Careers – Interview Questions That will Throw You for a Loop

http://editorial.careers.msn.com/articles/negtips
MSN Careers –Top 10 Tips for Successful Salary Negotiations

http://editorial.careers.msn.com/articles/salary/
MSN Careers –6 Steps to Handling Money Questions

http://editorial.careers.msn.com/articles/righttone/
MSN Careers –Set the Right Tone for Your Negotiations

http://editorial.careers.msn.com/articles/overview/
MSN Careers –The Listener Wins

http://editorial.careers.msn.com/articles/tips/
MSN Careers –Five Tips for Listening Well

BIBLIOGRAPHY

Collins, M. (1998). Network into marketing, advertising, and public relations careers. *National Association of Colleges and Employers*. 20-21.

Equal Opportunity Employment Journal. June 1998. Know the territory and dress accordingly. 8:9, 1-6.

Floyd, P.A. and Allen, B.J. (2008). *Professional Development for Pre-service Teachers,* 2nd ed. Boston: MA. Pearson Education.

Jeffries, P. (1998). If you don't have a job by graduation. *The Black Collegian.* 28:2 48-52.

Kaplan, R. (2003). Handling illegal questions. *Planning Job Choices: 2003*, 46th ed. National Association of Colleges and Employers 60-61.

Letourneau, T.M. (2003). Secrets to interview success. *Planning Job Choices 2003*, 46th ed. National Association of Colleges and Employers 56-57.

Muha, D. and Orgiefsky, R. (1995). The interview - The on-site visit. *Planning Job Choices: 1995*, College Placement Council, Inc.

Ryan, R. (2008). *Job Interviews: What to Wear*. www.robinryan.com.

Sabath, A.M. (2003). Dressing for the job. *Planning Job Choices: 2003, 46th ed*. National Association of Colleges and Employers, p. 66-67.

Shakoor, A. T. (2002). Typical on-campus interview questions. *The Black Collegian*. 33:1 70-71.

LABORATORY ACTIVITY 7.1

NAME _____ DATE _____

COURSE _____ SECTION _____

In small groups, discuss possible responses to the types of questions (Figures 7.1-7.5) that you might expect when interviewing for a teaching position. Hold mock interviews. Record your findings below.

LABORATORY ACTIVITY 7.2

NAME _____ DATE _____

COURSE _____ SECTION _____

Explore a variety of on-line sites related to the job interview. Generate a list of ten (10) sites not listed in the Web site section of the chapter. Complete and on-line resume. Use Laboratory 7.2 for your response.

CHAPTER 8

MARKETING YOURSELF: JOB SEARCH STRATEGIES AND THE APPLICATION PROCESS

"Every communication act is a message about you."
Anonymous

KEY CONCEPTS

1. The job search is an active process.
2. There are many sources for leads on job openings in your field.
3. The Internet can assist you in the job search process.
4. Networking is important to your job search.
5. There are seven types of letters that can be used in the job search process.

INTRODUCTION

You must actively seek job opportunities. In fact, you must work at finding a job and finding the right job will be frustrating at times. Employers are looking for people who truly want the job and will do a great job for them in return. You must be competitive in this competitive world if you want to work and to advance in your career in health, physical education and/or sport. Enthusiastic, creative, energetic, motivated, and directed individuals are easily identified and preferred by employers. Now it is time for you to develop your job search strategy to pursue your career goals. Get what you want and let the search process assist you, not defeat you.

YOUR JOB-SEARCH STRATEGY

Job-hunting is a full-time commitment. Thousands of job opportunities are advertised in newspapers and magazines daily. But you are not going to apply for every job advertised. You must select the jobs that are of interest to you. It is important to identify what you want before seeking it.

First you must ask these questions: "What kind of job do I want? How do I get it? Is the job in the right location? What type of salary must I have? Remember the most important question is to identify what you want before going after it.

Mullins stated, "Most job seekers suffer more from poor job-hunting skills than from lack of opportunity." He suggests that you "Make job hunting a full-time commitment." If you are unemployed, you should spend a minimum of 40 hours a week actively searching for work. As a full-time job seeker, your goal should be at least one contact a day with someone who has the power to hire you."

WHERE TO LOOK

Think…. If you were an employer and you were seeking employees where would you look for a job…? Be creative. Sources for looking for job opportunities in health, physical education and sport include:

Newspapers

Newspaper want ads, especially the Sunday newspaper, should be reviewed on a daily basis. Scan all ads; you never know where they may be listed. Read your local and neighborhood papers and papers from surrounding cities. Check specific sections of the newspaper.

- Under what other headings might a health position appear? List them in your journal.
- Under what other headings might a physical education position appear? List them in your journal.
- Under what other heading might a sport position appear? List them in your journal.

Job openings may be placed in the classified ads. Take your time in reading these ads. Check ads listed by corporations, organizations, school systems, and city, county and private employers.

Periodicals

Health, physical education and sport have numerous periodicals and publications. Many of these resources list job openings and, in addition, contain current information beneficial to individuals applying in these fields.

Publications such as: *Tips for Finding the Right Job* is a U.S. Department of Labor pamphlet offering advice on determining job skills, organizing the job search, writing a resume and interviewing. *Job Search Guide: Strategies for Professionals* is a U.S. Department of Labor publication that discusses specific steps job seekers should follow to identify employment opportunities

Other publications deal with more general topics and may contain an ad for your career. For example, magazines that deal with health and sports could contain such ads. Become familiar with a variety of specialty periodicals and periodicals that list only jobs. For example, *the National Employment Listing Service* contains only related employment opportunities. If you are interested in a federal job, the *Federal Jobs Register* is a valuable resource. For federal positions in and out of the country contact the U.S. Civil Service Commission. According to Krannich and Drannich, government agencies always hire, even during the worst of times. They have an average annual turnover rate of 10-14 percent. Federal agencies hire nearly 1,000 people each day, or 300,000 to 400,000 each year.

Internet

Using the Internet makes it easier to search for job openings in a variety of locations both in and out of the country daily. There are numerous Web sites that you can access to learn more about a specific organization, company, agency, community or even a school system. Furthermore, newspapers from across the country can be accessed over the Internet. Go online and search for school systems, agencies, organizations, companies or general locations that may be of interest to you.

Computer bulletin boards are popular ways of interacting with others having similar interests and for finding information about a particular topic. A computerized job network system, *America's Job Bank*, is run by the U.S. Department of Labor and lists approximately 50,000 job openings a week. Refer to the Web sites listed at the end of the chapter for additional sources.

Educational Institutions

University personnel offices often post job notices on a bulletin board, on a phone job line, in local newspapers, in organizational periodicals and newsletters, on the Internet, and other sources. Contact the personnel office on campus for a list of current openings. The Career Service Center is also a great resource on the university campus. Career Services have lists of positions available and reference libraries for further research. Additionally, they coordinate interviews with agencies looking to hire. Two or three times per year placement offices may sponsor career fairs for employers to interview for job opportunities.

Additional Places

The serious job hunter routinely contacts and or visits the city and or county school superintendent's personnel office; federal, state, county and municipal offices; local hospitals, community health centers; agencies such as the American Heart Association, American Red Cross, and American Diabetes Association regularly to check job postings and to find out what job openings are anticipated or available.

Check your local library for job listings and privately published services. Also, look in your local telephone directory. Check listings under government agencies (local, state and federal) for personnel departments. Employment services and organizations may also be able to assist you in finding jobs.

Unadvertised Jobs

Many jobs are not advertised and are actually filled before an ad is placed. It is your responsibility to learn about these. Active job seekers find job openings before the jobs are advertised by having established a relationship with the employer (as an intern or part time employee) and by making the employer aware of their interest before the job opening is posted. Advertisements for jobs run because of the department policy or to meet a legal obligation.

Telephone Inquiries

Telephone inquiries are an easy, quick, and nonthreatening way to ask if a certain department, agency, or company has, or expects, any job openings. Ask if a specific list of available jobs could be provide to you, or if you could be notified by phone or a mailer when a job opening occurs. With polite interaction, you may be able to get an individual notice from the contact person you impressed while inquiring about jobs. Also, ask if they know of anyone else who is hiring.

Personal Inquires

Employers are usually extremely busy and usually do not have or take time to visit with someone who has no appointment. If you use this risky approach, don't take up too much of their time. Always leave a resume even if you are not able to see anyone. Follow up with a letter, especially if someone took the time to talk with you. If you do get in to see the employer, deliver your message and get out in a few minutes. As a rule of thumb, if the employer looks at their watch, it is usually a sign that you need to state your case and soon leave. You do not want to aggravate a potential employer and as a result, get no job.

Networking

Networking is the process of connecting and interacting with individuals who can be helpful to you in your job search. Developing a network of contacts is the key to finding a job. You must constantly seek new contacts and possibilities if you want a job. Continue to expand your contacts even after you are hired. You never know when you may want or need to seek another job opportunity. Talk to anyone and everyone to establish contacts. For an example of a networking letter, refer to Figure 8.4 in this chapter.

"Networking 101," 1997 reports that approximately 70 percent of job openings are filled by people who heard about the job through word of mouth. The more contacts you have, the greater your odds are to be considered for a position. Mullins suggests: "Create a network of friendly contacts who can hire you or recommend you to others who can. As the saying goes, "it is not what you know but who you know or who knows you."

You are selling yourself. Take every opportunity to show yourself off in a positive and energetic way. Remember that you need only one YES, however you may have to struggle with many NOs along the way. Take every opportunity to make new contacts and to add to your contact list. You can use initial contacts and other contacts to add to your list. To develop your networking plan:

- Make initial contacts (company, school system, organization, agency name, address, phone, e-mail).
- Document the contacts (names/titles of contacts… ask for correct spelling if you are not for sure).
- Ask for additional contacts from the initial contact.
- Follow-up (1-2 weeks to contact or re-contact sources, follow-up each month afterward). Be an assertive applicant but not a bother to the employer.

CONTACTING PROSPECTIVE EMPLOYERS

You have searched a variety or sources to locate job opportunities that are of interest to you. Now you must make contact with those potential employers. You can use any one or all of the following methods to make contact.

U.S. Mail

Written material is a direct reflection of you as is the importance of appearance and making a good impression. Even though you may not actually see the person doing the hiring, if you supply a resume, chances are it will at least be reviewed. Have something of interest in your resume that reflects that you are the right person for the position.

Contacting prospective employers by mail is easy, quick and the most nonthreatening. However it is the least effective. It is easier to say no over the phone and with a letter than in person. With your resume always include a cover letter, which makes it more personal and sincere by introducing you and telling why you are writing. Refer to Chapter 5, cover letter. Writing skills are essential when you are trying to make a favorable impression. See tips for letter writing and job-search correspondence in this chapter.

E-Mail

Submitting your application electronically could be an excellent way to demonstrate your computer literacy. However, don't assume that all employers know how to retrieve your materials. Traditional employers/institutions might expect application materials to be sent in the traditional way. If you aren't sure whether it is appropriate, ask. Not every office is connected to the Internet and may not be capable of accessing e-mail and attachments.

Fax

Faxing provides the materials to the employer quickly, with a clean, mailed original to soon follow. Compared to e-mail, faxes do not look as good. If you fax, consider noting in your cover letter, submitted by fax and mail or e-mail. If you are not sure if fax is acceptable, ask. Most fax materials lose quality and even look cluttered. If you need to fax and do not own a machine, you can pay for this service at large secretarial services, office supply stores, and major hotels. Faxing should be used only if requested by the potential employer.

APPLYING FOR THE POSITION

You have found the job and now you have been asked to apply for the position. The first step usually involves completing an application form, taking test (teacher certification, health certification, etc.), and having a preliminary interview, background check, final interview and a medical exam. By having a copy of your resume with you, the application form should be simple procedure; however some forms are very complex.

If you are required to complete the application process on the spot, do it neatly using black ink. Write or print which ever is the most legibly. Think before you write so you will not have to erase, rewrite and cross out information. If there is something that you do not understand on the form, ask. If you are allowed to take the application form home, do so. Type your responses on the form neatly. Make several copies of the form and practice on it, therefore saving the original for the final draft.

Equal Employment Opportunity (EEO) guidelines make mandatory responses to questions about ethnic background, religious preference and marital status illegal, it is usually in your best interest to complete those optional sections, that is, if you want the job (See Chapter 10).

Today, many agencies and school systems are including a written essay as part of the application process. Candidates are requested to write two or three pages on a specific topic such as:

- Why did you select this career?
- Why have you selected this agency/organization/school system?
- Who are you? (Write a one-page autobiography.)

Tips For Submitting An Application For Employment

- If you do not type well, hire a professional.
- Application should be neat and easy to follow. Make sure entries in each block are in the block.
- Say you will accept the job. You can always decline.
- Never leave blocks blank. Give an answer, even it it's a "N/A."
- Collect all the information you need to complete the form (certificates, past work experiences, college transcripts, qualifications, etc.)
- Mail via Certified Mail and get a return receipt, or send information via Federal Express.
- Never leave gaps in documentation of employment dates.
- If you have teaching experience or administrative experience, explain concepts of your teaching skills and how well you managed, not how you did all of the work.
- You may send in lots and lots of application forms... Don't get discouraged... Be patient.

JOB SEARCH LETTERS

One of the most important but confusing aspects of finding a job is writing appropriate job-search letters. This may be the first time that you will have to compose and produce professional-level correspondence. You must meet the challenge of what to say and how to say it for a number of important, unfamiliar situations, such as applying for a job, expressing appreciation, and accepting or rejecting job offers. There is no single formula for a perfect letter that will work for every occasion, so you must give careful consideration and attention to detail in your writing. As an act of communication, your letters tell something about you as a responsible person with a positive attitude and as a prospective employee who knows how to function in a professional environment.

This section introduces you to the art of writing job-search correspondence. It entails general guidelines for producing high-quality letters, and samples of seven basic types of letters, and tips for letter writing. This information applies to hard copy (paper) and e-mail letters. Remember that every communication act is a message about you.

Tips For Letter Writing And Job-Search Correspondence

- Do all the writing yourself and take the responsibility for following up with employers.
- Always address your job-search letters to a specific individual with correct titles and business address.
- Use high-quality white or off-white bond paper and matching envelopes, of the usual business correspondence size, (8 2" x 11") for your hard copy letters.
- Use a word processor or typewriter. Type only on one side of the paper and keep it to one page.
- Provide a cover letter always with your resume.
- Keep the letter brief and to the point and avoid rehashing material from your resume.
- Letters should be neat in appearance and review for spelling, punctuation, English usage, form, etc. Remember to have an error free and clean copy final product.
- Design your letter to be work-centered, employer-centered, not self-centered. Your letter should address needs of employers and make the employers have a desire to learn more about you.
- Define the objectives of the letter and attempt to determine how these objectives can best be met. Generic, mass produced letters are ineffective.
- Avoid negative words, boastfulness, exaggeration, insincerity and inconsistency.
- Make your letters easy to read and always show appreciation to the employer for considering your application by granting you an interview.
- Be honest and always back up your correspondence with examples and evidence from your experience.
- Ask for assistance at your career services center.

Seven Basic Types of Letters

Communication skills are most important to bring to your career and your job-search letters will be the first samples employers will have of your competency. Your letters should be functional, understandable, easy to read, and pleasant in tone. Every communication act is a message about you and how you compose letters represents you. Skills in letter writing should be developed. If you need assistance contact the career advisor in your college, faculty or professionals in the selected career field. There are seven basic letters you may use during your job search. Each has its own function and should be used according to career and objectives. Be sure to sign the original and keep copies of all correspondence.

Networking Letter

This letter is designed to generate information interviews, not job interviews. It allows you to meet individuals who can give you specific information about your intended career. You are seeking information and your reasons for wanting to meet with a contact person must be sincere. Information interviewing, or "networking," requires preparation, sincerity and effort. The networking letter is the first step in the information interviewing process. See Figure 8.1.

Paragraph 1: Make a connection between you and the alumnus, your acquaintance, or anyone with a similar interest or background.

Paragraph 2: State your purpose without pressuring the person. Briefly explain your situation.

Paragraph 3: Request a meeting at a mutually convenient time and indicate that you will call to make arrangements. Usually a resume is not attached to a networking letter, but it may be presented during the interview to help the interviewer address your questions.

Figure 8.1   Networking Letter (Modified Block Format)

2118 Tanner Street
Tanner AFB, USA 09001
January 10, 2008

Ms. Courtney Zinke, Director
Shalimar Women's Life Center
13601 Shalimar Avenue
Sharlimar, FL 43011

Dear Ms. Zinke:

Dr. Pat Floyd, professor of physical education at Alabama State University, suggested that I contact you. She thought that you would be in an excellent position as an alumna to assist me with a career decision.

As a physical education student, I am exploring which career path to pursue. Athletics, sport management, sport communication, the fitness industry, and teaching work all sound interesting to me at this point, but I want to go into my campus interviews next semester with a clear sense of direction. I would like to get your advice on the long-term career implications of each path as well as a better handle on the day-to-day activities of a fitness/wellness manager.

I shall call you next week to see if we can arrange a brief meeting at your convenience. Thank you for considering my request.

Sincerely,

(Written signature)
Elizabeth A. Williams

Prospecting Letter

The purposes of this letter are to prospect for potential vacancies in your career, to get your resume read, and to generate interviews. Prospecting letters are used extensively for long-distance searches. Target specific individuals in specific organizations. Use position information; focus on broader career and /or organizational dimensions to describe how your qualifications match the work environment. See Figure 8.2.

Figure 8.2   Prospecting Letter (Modified Block Format)

207 Opothleohola Street
Wetumpka, AL 35929
February 26, 2008

Mr. Zachary A. Zinke
Director of Health Promotions
Taylor Mercantile Company
Shalimar, FL 46932

Dear Mr. Zinke:

I read your company's open position in *The Journal of Physical Education, Recreation & Dance* and would like to inquire about employment opportunities in your management-training program. I want to work in wellness centers and would like to relocate to the Shalimar area after graduation.

I will receive my B. S. degree in fitness/sport management studies this May. My interest in fitness started in junior high intramural sports and developed further through a variety of volunteer and work experiences during college. My internship with K-12 students convinced me to pursue a career in wellness. When I researched the top wellness centers in Shalimar, Taylor Mercantile Company emerged as having an excellent market position, excellent fitness program for their employees, and a reputation for excellent customer service for the community. In short, you provide the kind of professional environment I seek.

My resume is enclosed for your consideration. My education and experience match the qualifications you seek in your employees, but they don't tell the whole story. I know from evaluations from my instructors at Alabama State University I have the interpersonal skills and motivation needed to build a successful career in fitness/wellness management. My relatively extensive experience gave me confidence in my career direction and in my abilities to perform competently.

I know how busy you must be during this time of year, but I would appreciate a few minutes of your time. I shall call you during the week of February 15 to discuss employment possibilities. In the meantime, if you need to contact me, my number is 850-386-0000 and my e-mail is m-holman@alabamastateuniversity.edu.

Thank you very much for considering my request. I look forward to talking with you.

Sincerely,

(Written signature)

Melissa A. Holman

Application letter

An application letter is often the first contact between you and the employer. Research the organization before you begin to write in order to make a good first impression. The application letter is to get your enclosed resume read and to get those interviews. Use this type of letter to inquire about specific job advertisements and apply for vacancies that are known. Keep the letter sales-oriented and indicate your main qualifications. The main function of an application letter is to entice the employer's interest in you so your resume will be read. Develop one basic letter, which can be changed slightly for different positions. Your letter should be personal but follow a standard business format. Identify and send the application letter to the person who is doing the hiring. Structure your application letters with three or four paragraphs. See Figure 8.3.

Paragraph 1: Reveal your purpose and interests. Identify the position and your source of information (school placement office, newspaper ad, faculty referral, etc.) Introduce your themes.

Paragraph 2: Outline your strongest qualifications that match the position requirements. Provide evidence of your related experiences and accomplishments. Make reference to your enclosed resume.

Paragraph 3: Sell your personal qualities and motivation to perform well in the position.

Paragraph 4: Suggest an action plan. Request an interview and indicate that you will call during a specific time period to discuss interview possibilities. Show appreciation to the reader for his/her time and consideration.

Figure   8.3   Application Letter (Full Block Format)

3004 Alford Avenue
Rutledge, AL 36071
January 15, 2008

Dr. Earl L. Dees
Manager of Life Health Center
Life Health Center
3001 Crawford Lane
Pensacola, FL 30521

Dear Dr. Dees:

I am applying for the position of exercise health/fitness specialist that was advertised on December 12 with the placement service at Alabama State University. The position seems to fit very well with my education, experience, and career interests.

Your position requires skills and experience in health and fitness, with an educational background in health, physical education and sports, computer systems, exercise/fitness applications software, and group exercise. With a major in health and physical education, I have training in fitness activities that include group exercise for adults as well as the older adult. I have served as a volunteer in the local hospital wellness center, assisted in organizing programs/speakers for the state professional organization's health and fitness conferences and gained valuable experience in microcomputers and a variety of software programs at the local hospital wellness center. My practical experience in the university's health, physical education and sports department as an office assistant, assistant in the school's intramural sports programs and a student assistant to the aerobic and exercise physiology labs have given me valuable exposure to the health/fitness profession. Additionally, I worked as a student intern in the K-12 levels and served as a volunteer in the after school sports programs where I gained knowledge of teaching and sport activities. My enclosed resume provides more details on my qualifications.

My background and career goals seem to match your job requirements well. I am confident that I can perform the job effectively. Furthermore, I am genuinely interested in the position and in working for the Life Health Center. Your agency has an excellent reputation and comes highly recommended to me.

Would you please consider my request for a personal interview to discuss further my qualifications and to learn more about this opportunity? I shall call you next week to see if a meeting can be arranged. Should you need to reach me, please feel free to call me at 334-300-0000 or w-dean@alabamastateuniversity.edu. If I am not in, please leave a message on my answering machine or e-mail me and I will reply within a day.

Thank you for your consideration. I look forward to talking with you.

Sincerely yours,

(Written signature)

Reed D. Zinke

Thank You Letter

This is one of the least used tools in a job search, yet one of the most important. A thank-you letter is a professional courtesy as well as a method of establishing communication with the employer. It is used to establish goodwill, to express appreciation, and/or strengthen your candidacy. Everyone who assists you in any way gets a thank-you letter. Thank you letters should be sent within two or three days to everyone who interviewed you. The letters should be only two or three paragraphs in length and your letters should be warm and personal. Use them as an opportunity to:

- Reemphasize your strongest qualifications
- Reiterate your interest in a position
- Provide supplemental information not previously given
- Bring attention to your qualifications and the job requirements
- Express your sincere appreciation

In addition, thank-you letters should be sent to each of your contacts who granted you information interviews and to people who provided references for you. See Figure 8.4.

Figure 8.4 Thank-You Letter (Modified Block Format)

3004 Sam Snead Court.
Pace, FL 34587
April 6, 2008

Mr. Glenn O. Rose
Sports Information Director
WITZ Television
Montgomery, AL 34501

Dear Mr. Rose:

I want to thank you very much for interviewing me yesterday for the associate sports marketing director's position. I enjoyed meeting you and learning more about your television program and work.

My enthusiasm for the position and my interest in working for WITZ were strengthened as a result of the interview. I think my education and cooperative education experiences fit nicely with the job requirements, and I'm sure that I could make a significant contribution to WITZ over time.

I want to reiterate my strong interest in the position and in working with you and your staff. You provide the kind of opportunity I seek. Please feel free to call me at 271-450-0000 or e-mail me @ c-zinke @ aol.com if I can provide you with any additional information.

Again, thank you for the interview and your consideration.

                Sincerely,

                (Written signature)

                M. Colton Zinke

Acceptance Letter

This letter is used to accept the employment; restate position classification, compensation offered, medical examinations, travel plans, and the starting date if previously established. Often the acceptance letter follows a telephone conversation during which the details of the offer and the terms of employment are discussed. The letter confirms your acceptance of the offer, expresses your appreciation for the opportunity, and positively reinforces the employer's decision to hire you. Express your appreciation. Do not delay. Procrastination makes a bad impression. See Figure 8.5.

Figure 8.5   Acceptance Letter (Full Block)

---

321 Hemp Street
Portland, OR 52346
May 3, 2008

Mr. Jim Thompson, Director
Sport Communication Department
Alabama State University
604 Alabama Avenue
Montgomery, AL 35607

Dear Mr. Thompson:

I am writing to confirm my acceptance of your employment offer of May 5 and to tell you how delighted I am to be joining Alabama State University. The work is exactly what I have prepared to perform and hoped to do. I feel confident that I can make a significant contribution to the university, and I am grateful for the opportunity you have given me.

As we discussed, I will report to work at 7:30 a.m. on June 3 and will have completed the medical examination and drug testing by the start date. Additionally, I shall complete all employment and insurance forms for the new employee orientation on June 15.

I look forward to working with you and your fine team. I appreciate your confidence in me and am very happy to be joining your staff.

Sincerely,

(Written signature)

Darrell E. Walker

Withdrawal Letter

Once you have accepted a position, you have an ethical obligation to inform all other employers of your decision and to withdraw your employment application from consideration. Your withdrawal letter should express appreciation for the employer's consideration and courtesy. It may be appropriate to state that your decision to go with another organization was based on you having the job to fit you better at this stage in your career. Do not say that you obtained a better position. See Figure 8.6.

Figure 8.6   Withdrawal Letter (Full Block Format)

8004 Scott Street
Dallas, Texas 27012
June 6, 2008

Dr. Linda E. Ramsey, Director
The Sports Marketing Corporation
6661 Holly Street
Washington, NC 27104

Dear Dr. Ramsey:

I am writing to inform you that I am withdrawing my application for the program manager position with the corporation. As I indicated in my interview with you, I have been exploring several employment possibilities. This week I was offered an administrative position with a local, city government, and recreation department and, after careful consideration, I decided to accept it. The position provides a very good match for my interests at this point in my career.

I want to thank you very much for interviewing and considering me for your position. I enjoyed meeting you and learning about the innovative company programs you are planning. You have a fine corporation and I wish you and your staff well.

Sincerely,

(Written signature)

Kalilah I. Allen

Rejection Letter

Candidates as well as employers send rejections of offers. The purpose of this letter is to decline employment offers that do not fit their career objectives and interests. Express your appreciation for the offer and for the organization's interest in you when declining the offer of employment. Indicate that you have carefully considered the offer and have decided not to accept it. Be sure to thank the employer for the offer and for consideration of you as a candidate. See Figure 8.7.

Figure 8.7   Rejection Letter (Block Format)

2601 East .Lee Street
Glenwood, CA 52261
July 8, 2008

Ms. Jean Thompson
Director of Sales
Thompson Sports Chain
Greenville, AL 45608

Dear Ms. Thompson:

Thank you very much for offering me the position of sales with Thompson Sports Chain. I appreciate your discussing the details of the position with me and giving me time to consider your offer.

You have a fine organization and there are many aspects of the position, which are very appealing to me. However, I believe it is in our mutual best interest that I decline your kind offer. This has been a difficult decision for me, but I believe it is the appropriate one for my career at this time.

I want to thank you for the consideration and courtesy given to me. It was a pleasure meeting you and your fine staff.

Sincerely,

(Written signature)

Huriah Stroud

References Available Upon Request

References are from individuals who can discuss your skills and attributes for a particular job.
When an employer asks for references it generally indicates that you are being considered for the position. It is important that you select people who can provide the information the employer is seeking. Your reference list should contain information for three to five individuals. Lists references on a separate sheet from your resume and include key contact information such as: name, title/position, and complete mailing address, phone number and e-mail address (if appropriate). Don't mail your reference list with your resume and cover letter unless specified. Bring it with you to the interview. Select the right people to help you secure a job offer. When selecting references, consider the following:

- Does the person know you well and as a professional? This person should know you better so they can discuss your skills using more specific examples. Avoid using personal references such as mom, dad, and neighbors. You need this person to discuss your skills and abilities rather than your personality.
- Will this person help you get the job by providing a positive recommendation? Select a person who would offer positive comments about you. Consider asking individuals from part-time/full-time jobs, volunteer experiences, academic advisers, supervisors from internships, and student group advisers to serve as references.

Tips for References

- Inform your references of your career plans and the types of positions that you are applying.
- Provide a copy of your resume. It gives the complete picture of who you are and what you have accomplished.
- Contact your references after the interview when an employer asks for your reference list. That way, your references can expect contact with the employer.
- Keep your references informed of your job-search progress. Inform them when you accept a position and don't forget to thank them for their assistance.
- Stay in touch because you may need to call them again for another job.

REJECTION BY PROSPECTIVE EMPLOYER

"No, we have chosen another candidate for the position. Thank you for applying." None of us likes to hear this from a potential employer, especially after you have spent numerous days/weeks, time and energy pursuing this job. Get used to it! You will inevitably receive a certain number of rejections during your job search process and career.

Job searching is risk-taking. A rejection does not have to be taken as a failure. Rejection may be a positive process in disguised. There may be several reasons for being rejected for a position. For example, the employer did not feel that you were right for the department/school/agency or the position was already filled before you even applied. Being rejected from one job may mean a grand opportunity for another. It is important to remember that you need to plan your days, set hours including breaks, take several days off to regroup, plan time with people who you like and like you, seek a support group, and share ideas, hints with others with and without jobs. Review your strategy and continue to plan and follow-up. Continue to build your networking system; the next contact could have the right job for you.

SUMMARY

Remember that you and your situation in selecting a career are unique. Never wait for a job; you must work at finding the job. Identify what you want to do before pursuing it. Now it is time to make the job hunting process a full-time commitment, spending a minimum of 40 hours a week actively searching for the job of your dreams. If you are having problems with your written communication, perhaps you need to do more foundational work in clarifying your career direction and in articulating your value to potential employers.

Showing your individuality can be expressed through your writing by convincing the employer of your value as a prospective employee and to persuade the employer to take action in your favor. Through practice you can develop your writing skills that will enhance your career and skill of writing. It is important to remember that effective communication rest with the writer, not with the reader. The job search process involves your time, effort, diligence and commitment. Network any opportunity that may present itself and always follow up a contact with a thank you. By taking this process seriously you can find the job that is self-gratifying to you in the years ahead.

REFLECTIONS

1. In small groups, discuss and list as many sources that you can in which employment ads may appear. List 10 contacts you have available right now through which you could establish your networking contacts. Use Laboratory 8.1 for your response.

2. Explore a variety of on-line sites related to the job search process. Generate a list of five (5) sites not listed in the Web Feature section of the chapter. Use Laboratory 8.2 for your response.

WEB SITES

www.jobweb.com
The Art of Writing Job-Search Letters

http://career-advice.monster.com/resume-tips/home.aspx?WT.srch=1
Career Advice

http://www.careerpath.com
Career Path

www.employmentspot.com/employment-tips
Employment Tips

www.bumnomore.com
Job Search Strategies

www.edataintegrityreport.com/images/MarketingYourself.pdf
Marketing Yourself in a Job Search

www.quintcareers.com/networking_guide.html
Networking Your Way to a New Job

http://hotjobs.yahoo.com
Yahoo Hot Jobs

www.monster.com
Your Calling is Calling

www.totaljobs.com/content/Applications/Personalmarketingcampaign.html
Your Personal Marketing Campaign

BIBLIOGRAPHY

Bardwell, C. B. (1998). How to evaluate a job offer. *The Black Collegian*. 28:2. 64-68.

Floyd, P. A. and Allen, B. J. (2008). *Professional Preparation of Pre-Service Teachers,* 2nd ed. Boston, MA: Pearson Education.

Harr, J. S. and Hess, K. M. (2005). *Careers in Criminal Justice and Related Fields: From Internship to Professionalism,* 5th ed. Belmont, CA: Wadsworth/Thomson Learning.

Networking 101. (1997). *Career Path Coach*, 1, 10.

U.S. Civil Service Commission, 1900 East Street, NW, Washington, DC 20006.

LABORATORY ACTIVITY 8.1

NAME _____ DATE _____

COURSE _____ SECTION _____

In small groups, discuss and list as many sources as you can in which employment ads may appear. List 10 contacts you have available right now through which you could establish your networking contacts. Use Laboratory 8.1 for your response.

LABORATORY ACTIVITY 8.2

NAME _____ DATE _____

COURSE _____ SECTION _____

Explore a variety of on-line sites related to the job search process. Generate a list of five (5) sites not listed in the Web Site section of the chapter. Use Laboratory 8.2 for your response.

CHAPTER 9

BEGINNING YOUR CAREER

"Preparation for the future is critical because that's where you'll be spending
the rest of your life!"

Anonymous

KEY CONCEPTS

1. The first year is a critical period in a new career.
2. The manner in which you enter an organization is key to your success.
3. A professional is committed to the profession and to contributing to the profession.
4. Office dynamics impact what goes on in the workplace.

INTRODUCTION

You have achieved a milestone in your life. You have successfully completed those critical steps leading to your new career. You completed your college education, developed and impressively implemented your resume writing and interviewing skills, and celebrated a very significant achievement – you got your first position as a professional. And now it's time to go to work. This marks a new beginning with a whole new set of challenges.

Today is the first day of your professional career. Remember that this is a unique day and you will never have another day like today. Wear the suit that you know makes you look good. First impressions do count and if you feel confident, you'll look confident to others. Eat breakfast before you leave home, fresh breath and clean teeth are a must. Be sure to leave plenty of time to get to work early.

When you arrive at your new workplace take a deep breath and walk in with a smile on your face. Keep your head up and remember to make eye contact. Be polite and friendly to everyone, whether it's the receptionist, the custodian, your colleagues, your subordinates, or your new supervisor. As you go through the day, introduce yourself to those individuals that you encounter and to whom you have not been introduced.

THE CRITICAL FIRST YEAR

Every year, thousands of college students successfully find employment in the career of their choice. They begin work with great energy and enthusiasm, only to find disappointment. Many of them find that work is a different world and they don't know "how to go to work". They don't understand what it takes to successfully enter an organization for the first time.

The first year in your new career is a period of transition. It is both a unique and a critical period. It is unique because you will never again have another first year of your professional career. It is unique because you're not a college student but you're not a full professional either. It is also unique because it is a distinct stage in your career that can critically affect your success within the organization and possibly the future success of your career. Research shows that your approach to your first year will not only affect your success within the organization, but it will have a major impact on your future salary, career satisfaction, and your personal feelings about success and commitment to your career.

Entering a New Organization

A successful career should begin with a successful first year. The manner in which you enter the organization is key to that success. It is important to enter with the appropriate expectations and attitudes.
Many new employees become frustrated after a short time in their new career because their expectations are not met. Most likely many things about your job won't be what you expected them to be. You won't receive the kind of attention from your colleagues that you received while being recruited. Your job won't be as important, as glamorous, or as high level as you thought. And you won't be able to show your individual talents because collaboration and teamwork are much more important than individual accomplishments. The pressure of the job, the extra hours of work, and the types of assignments may be very different from what you expected. The solution is to keep your expectations in check - keep them realistic. Initially it is essential that you:

- Learn the culture

- Earn respect and credibility

- Establish yourself

Learn the culture

The culture of an organization can loosely be defined as its personality. The culture is manifested in the behavior of employees who adhere to a unique set of values and norms that are often informal and unspoken. You must learn and understand the culture of the organization. Pay attention to the way things are done. Observe those around you. How do they behave? What do they spend their time doing? How do they communicate? How do they work together? It is important that you know what is expected of you, particularly the accepted work ethic and social norms. All these things are a part of the culture and they are unwritten. To learn them you have to pay attention.

Failure to understand the culture will almost assure that you will make many embarrassing and avoidable mistakes that will damage your career. While it's okay to hold onto and use some of the things you learned previously, remember that every workplace has it's own way of doing things. Never say "that's not how we did it at my old job" or tell supervisors or senior colleagues how they should be doing something. While innovation is a good thing, walking in and talking about "better ways" to do things, will likely be met with negative reactions. Why? First, you know very little, if anything, about why they do things the way they do. Second, you haven't gained the trust of your colleagues. Finally, people, by nature, are threatened by change. Acting as if you "know it all" is a sure way to destroy relationships with experienced colleagues and you may never recover from the mistake.

Take time to learn the system. By observing and listening you will learn about your environment, your job, and the people you work with. Observe, study, and learn how things are done and by whom. In addition, become familiar with the facilities, tools, and resources available to you. While you are learning the culture, go by the book. Be sure to observe all company policies and follow proper business etiquette.

Earn respect and credibility

Earning respect and credibility is essential for a successful career. Your peers, subordinates, and supervisors are all watching and attempting to assess your ability to succeed. You want to establish your reputation as a competent and valued employee, worthy of their respect. How do you do this? The first thing that you must realize is that you get respect by giving respect. As a new employee, you will get more respect from your colleagues if you show respect for them. During your first weeks and after, show your colleagues that you respect their experience and expertise.

Feel free to ask questions. Everything is new and there is much for you to learn. Be open to learning about your work and about the broader organization. People generally like to help others, and it usually makes them feel good about themselves and about you. Be open and accept offers of help, especially if you need it. If you refuse all offers of help your colleagues may get the impression that you are a snob or a "know it all" and some may decide that they will not help you in the future. This is not to say that you should act as if you know nothing. If you are asked for your opinion, give it. If you need to make a decision, make it. Show sincere interest and a desire to learn. Many of your experienced colleagues have a great deal to offer. Give them the opportunity to share their knowledge and skills with you.
Credibility is earned over time. Since you are a new employee with no track record, your credibility good judgment, positive relationships with colleagues, and willingness to change and learn will go far in establishing your credibility. According to Holton, your colleagues are looking for an attitude that shows confidence in your potential but humility about what you can do from the beginning. They want to see that your expectations are realistic, that you are willing to work hard to learn how to make a contribution, that you recognize your role as a new employee, and that you are willing to do what it takes to earn respect and credibility. Show initiative, be productive, make suggestions respectfully, and work hard.

Your colleagues will respond to you differently, work with you differently, and judge you differently. You have to approach them differently in response. Holton suggests that you learn the art of being new and understand the importance of this highly significant transition period. Accept the role of "new kid on the block" and spend your energy on learning the organization and gaining acceptance. It takes time to understand and earn the rights, responsibilities, and credibility of a professional. You will have to "pay your dues" just as everyone else has while you earn your respect and credibility.

Establish yourself

Many of your early career opportunities will depend on the impressions you make on the people you work with and their perceptions of you. The natural tendency is to try to establish yourself by showing how smart and talented you are as fast as you can. To make a good impression you offer what you think are some great ideas for change and you try to make important contributions, only to find that your ideas weren't that great after all and what's worse is nobody is listening. A better approach to making a good impression is to demonstrate the maturity to know how much you don't know. This means observing your colleagues, learning the organization, understanding how things are done, and earning acceptance as a member of the team before you expect to make intelligent suggestions for change or have your ideas accepted. If you are successful, you will be given opportunities to make real contributions to the organization. If you then take advantage of these early opportunities by demonstrating how smart and talented you are, more opportunities to succeed will follow. If you are not successful during this period, you will be labeled as immature and relegated to less significant assignments. Although an entire career is not necessarily totally ruined in the first few months to a year, it can take years to recover from a bad start. The following are some strategies for establishing yourself and making a successful transition into the workplace:

- Work smarter, harder, faster - continually seek ways to function more effectively and efficiently; do what needs to be done, do it right and do it on time,

- Adapt to change – change is inevitable and it is constant, see it as an opportunity to grow and learn,

- Document value-added – find appropriate ways to contribute and document the work that you do; when asked or when it is appropriate, inform your supervisor of your achievements,

- Look for leadership opportunities – be willing and able to assume a leadership role when the opportunity arises, use this to demonstrate your abilities and value to the organization,

- Communicate openly and directly – communication is essential to success in every work environment, the way you communicate reflects how you perceive and perform your job.

PROFESSIONALISM

The term professional is a noun identifying one as engaged in a profession. It is also an adjective describing one as worthy of the high standard of a profession and as exhibiting a high level of knowledge and skills. A professional is committed to the profession and to developing into a contributing member of the profession. Buley describes the professional as one whom:

- **Has good communication skills** - part of being professional is how well one communicates in both oral and written forms,

- **Gives quality performance** - the skills of the profession are performed at a very high level,

- **Is predictable and consistent** - being a professional involves reliability and commitment to completing the job,

- **Is self-motivated, self-reliant and takes responsibility** - this is a self-starter who gets things done and doesn't expect others to do their work,

- **Works well under pressure** - the quality of work is even higher when the pressure is on,

- **Is always willing to learn** - education does not stop at graduation, professional development continues throughout professional life,

- **Understands interconnectedness with humanity** - because all that we do impacts others, we must behave ethically.

Parkay and Stanford define professionalism as having three dimensions: professional behavior, lifelong learning and involvement in the profession. Professional behavior indicates a commitment to professional practice and ethical standards. Lifelong learning signifies a commitment to professional growth. Involvement indicates participation in the profession on a broader scale.

Professional Behavior

When you begin working in your new career you will be expected to perform as a professional. You will be expected to know the basics and, more than likely, no one will take the time to ask if you do. It would be extremely disappointing to lose your job because you don't know what the situation demands. You must have some idea of what to expect and what the situation demands in order to be successful and to keep your job.

One place to begin is with your interpersonal skills. It is essential that you work well with others and that you are sensitive to their feelings and needs. You must develop and maintain a good relationship with supervisors, colleagues, and subordinates and understand what they expect of you. Seek to develop a good rapport with your supervisor from the start. In your first meeting, get a clear understanding of what your supervisor expects of you, your specific responsibilities, how your job fits into the overall mission and strategy of the organization, the scope of your authority, and who has authority to give you assignments. Ask for feedback and constructive criticism to help you learn to be more effective.

Meet your colleagues and subordinates on a warm and personal level. Show that you are a team player by working to develop rapport and supportive relationships with them. Be consistent in your behavior and style to allow others to become accustomed to your personality. Refrain from making criticisms about the job or other employees in public. Be patient and learn to listen to those around you. Keep a sense of humor but make sure that it is appropriate humor. Treat others and their experience with respect.

Dependability is a significant element of professionalism. It is highly important that you can be counted on. Be aware of your limits and don't take on more than you can handle. Complete projects, reports, and assignments promptly. Don't abuse leave time. Arrive for work, meetings, and appointments on time. Do whatever you say you will do and do it when you say you will do it.

Compatibility is also important. Participate in social activities so other can get to know you but maintain discretion in the amount of socializing on work time. Avoid office politics but understand that they are very much a part of the culture. Keep away from confrontations with supervisors and colleagues. And avoid disrespectful and offensive behavior.

Avoiding Offensive Behavior

It is important to remember proper etiquette. People may not remember your politeness, but they certainly will remember rude behavior. Disrespectful and offensive behavior in the workplace is not an uncommon occurrence. Strangely enough, many people don't realize that they are being disrespectful or that they are exhibiting offensive behavior. Risqué and off color jokes and stories are often prime examples of offensive behavior. They have no place in the workplace, especially one with which you are unfamiliar. You don't know your colleagues' personalities well enough to know what reactions these jokes and stories will engender. You can avoid offending your colleagues by becoming cognizant of your actions and making a concerted effort to shun those that are or that just might be offensive. The following actions are likely to be offensive to your colleagues.

- **Neglecting to use common courtesies:**

  - Not saying "please" and "thank you"
  - Taking supplies from co-workers' desk without permission
  - Leaving common work and break areas in disarray after you use them
  - Having loud phone conversations
  - Chewing gum loudly

- **Neglecting to use professional courtesies:**

  - Showing up late for meetings
  - Entering someone's office without knocking
  - Looking at colleague's computer screen over his/her shoulder
  - Talking behind someone's back
  - Asking a colleague to lie for you
  - Blaming someone else when you are at fault
  - Taking credit for someone else's work
  - Asking a subordinate to do something unrelated to work (run errands)
  - Publicly complaining about the organization, supervisor, or colleague
  - Opening a colleague's mail
  - Not pulling your own weight

- **Other offensive behaviors:**

  - Having a condescending attitude toward others
  - Wearing too much perfume or cologne
  - Taking the last of something without replacing it
  - Espousing your political or religious beliefs
  - Sending unwanted mail, including email
  - Smoking in common areas
  - Telling offensive jokes

It may not be easy for new employees to know exactly what appropriate behavior is. But, if you take a conservative, low-key approach and observe those around you who have been around for a while, you will be able to determine what is appropriate and what is not. Additionally, use your common sense. Taking a quiet, low-key and common sense approach you will experience less difficulty in adjusting to your new role.

Accepting Criticism

Beginning a new career means that you will face many new challenges. As you attempt to meet these challenges it is inevitable that you will make mistakes. This is to be expected. Considering that most people learn from their mistakes, you should regard your mistakes as learning opportunities. The hardest part of this may be having someone tell you that you have done something wrong and accepting the criticism. How you handle constructive criticism is often a critical part of formal and informal evaluation. Failure to respond appropriately can negatively affect your success on your new job.

It is essential that you accept constructive criticism in a mature and professional manner and that you process the information. Ask questions if you are unsure. Admit to and learn from your mistakes and accept suggestions for improvement. Hopefully this will prevent or, at least, decrease the reoccurrence of the same or similar mistakes and contribute to your overall improvement. Getting angry, arguing, challenging your supervisor, or complaining to colleagues might well cost you your job.

On occasion, unfair and unwarranted criticisms occur as a result of personality conflicts, illegal discrimination, or harassment. If you genuinely feel that you are being harassed or treated improperly, continue to respond maturely and professionally. Talk with the person first. If you cannot resolve things on this level, then proceed up the chain of command to address the problem. See Chapter 10 for details on discrimination issues.

The Unexpected

In a days work, any number of little crises may crop up in the workplace. Being prepared for these difficulties is important both to the well-being of the organization and to your job success. The employee who solves a problem that threatens productivity will certainly be looked upon favorably. As you learn the organization, look for potential problem situations and formulate a plan that could ease the crisis. These plans will not prevent the unpredictable, but they will help you be prepared to act quickly and competently.

Professional Dress

What do your clothes say about you? Do people form opinions about you based on the way you dress? You can bet that they do. Unless you work in a job that requires a uniform, choosing clothes for work can be difficult. What do you wear? You want to be a success; you have to dress for it. Research your office environment. Every office is different. Fashion, advertising, education, and the arts often allow more creativity; while law and accounting lean toward conformity.

You may have the opportunity to work in an environment where accepted dress requirements are more relaxed. Looking neat should be a priority. Even if the dress code is more relaxed, you should still look professional. This does not mean that you must avoid any sense of individuality in the workplace. However, let common sense prevail when dressing for work. Obviously, some types of clothing are inappropriate for certain work environments. In addition, some organizations have a dress code that all employees are required to follow. Sometimes you won't find these dress codes in writing; but if you observe those around you you'll find that all employees are dressed in a similar way. What ever you do, project your professional image. In addition, keep this rule in mind - if what you wear is distracting to others you shouldn't wear it to work. See Chapter 7 for details on appropriate dress.

Lifelong Learning

Lifelong learning is an essential commitment necessary for continued success and advancement in your career. The world of work constantly changes. One of the consequences of change is having to continually expand or refine your base of knowledge and skills. Your level of competence is greatly affected by your willingness to continue to grow professionally through continued education and study. Set high standards for yourself. Continue to improve your skills, especially in oral and written communication and technology. Learn as much as possible. Take advantage of courses and workshops offered or financed by the organization and professional associations. Employers are more likely to retain and promote employees who upgrade their knowledge and skills over those who do not.

Finding a mentor is another way to continue your learning. According to many experts, anyone who is beginning a new career and hopes to have a successful career should participate in a mentor/protégé relationship. A mentor is an individual who possesses the wisdom that only experience can provide. The protégé is someone who is looking for career success and advancement. The relationship benefits both mentor and protégé. The protégé receives guidance and helpful advice. The mentor benefits from the opportunity to strengthen leadership skills.

Mentoring relationships may be formal or informal. Many companies have programs for matching new employees with those already established in their jobs. Many professional associations have mentoring programs available and you may also fine mentors via the Internet. It is important to choose a mentor whose goals are similar to your own who is on the same career path. Choose a mentor who has time to give to the relationship. Likewise, you must find the time to participate. As the one who will benefit most, you must make the initial step in establishing contact with a potential mentor. You must also work to maintain the relationship.

Involvement in the Profession

A major component of your development as a professional is involvement in the profession. Membership and participation in professional associations is a primary vehicle for that involvement and is often considered a measure of professional commitment. Membership provides an opportunity for you to become involved in your career on a broader scale. There is a professional association for almost any career field and you can join at any time. Professional associations provide a number of services to members including:

- Publications (journals and newsletters)
- Job listings
- Consultant resource lists
- Courses and seminars
- Conferences/conventions

Your involvement should begin while you are a student and continue throughout your professional career.
Many academic departments and colleges sponsor student professional associations. Membership in the student associations will provide opportunities for you to work with fellow professional students to plan and implement activities, enhance your educational and recreational experiences, mentor underclass majors, provide services for the university and the community, and link to the local, state, district, and/or national associations. Your membership and active participation in the student association demonstrates that you value your chosen profession and you believe that it is important. Many professional associations have substantially reduced membership fees for college students.

Membership and active participation in local, state, district and national professional associations provides a multitude of opportunities. Active participation includes attending conferences/conventions, volunteering to work on committees and in leadership positions, making presentations at conferences/conventions, and contributing to the field. Attending conferences/conventions allows you to meet the leaders in your field, receive information on the latest developments in the field as well as their application to practical situations, make professional and personal contacts, learn about career opportunities and much more.

Volunteering to work on committees and in leadership positions allows you to serve your profession, to understand how your professional association works and to prepare you for other leadership roles. Making presentations at conferences and publishing in the association journal or newsletter allows you to share your knowledge and expertise with others in the profession. You can check with your major advisor or the staff at your career services center for on-campus and local chapters of professional associations. You may also use the directory of *National Trade & Professional Associations* or the Internet to research professional associations.

OFFICE DYNAMICS

The dynamics among those in the workplace play an import role in the interactions and relationships between colleagues. It is inevitable that you will encounter a variety of things that may not necessarily be work related; however, they greatly impact what goes on in the workplace. Office politics, gossip, and other intangibles have a presence in most, if not every workplace. To be successful, you will have to learn how to cope with the circumstances.

Office Politics and the Grapevine

Every organization has its politics. Office politics is something that most people recognize when they see it, but find difficult to define. Webster's defines politics as "competition between interest groups or individuals for power and leadership in a government or other group; while Alesko defines it as "the use and misuse of power in the workplace." Office politics is not always a bad thing. However, as a new employee you don't know where the political lines are drawn and its complexities may be so deep that you can get caught up in it before you realize it.

A 1998 study by Accuountemps reported that office politics is an increasing problem with 18 percent of administrator's time spent resolving resulting conflicts among employees. Besides causing problems for colleagues who work together, politics can distract employees attention their jobs causing financial loss by the organization and, in turn, loss of jobs.

Office politics can be highly competitive with extremely high stakes. To succeed, you must know the rules. Succeed and you get the better assignments, get promoted, or more importantly keep your job. Lose and you may be stuck with insignificant assignments, overlooked for promotions, or looking for a new job. Harr and Hess suggest that to understand politics, you must recognize that politics are impossible to understand. They go so far as to say that "Politics can be a deadly game and should be avoided." However, office politics may not be totally avoidable. You may have to learn to cope with it, and in doing so, be particularly careful.

The grapevine is closely related to office politics. And like office politics, is an unavoidable presence in every workplace. McKay suggests that the grapevine be considered the unofficial office newsletter. It is important to pay attention to what is being said. You can gain valuable insight into office dynamics, colleagues' personalities, and other bits of useful information. However, it is important not to contribute to the grapevine. This holds especially true when you are new. You don't want to begin your career with a reputation for being a gossip.

The grapevine can have two faces, one negative and one positive. Gossip that is damaging or that spreads false information is negative and is unwelcome. Watch out for the office troublemaker. Every office has one. This is the gossip that comes up to you and says something like: "The boss is always nice to new employees. Wait til you've been here a while." The office troublemaker is the one who tends to stir up trouble and then pretends to have nothing to do with it. Listen to what this person tells you, there may be some truth to it, but it may be greatly exaggerated.

Some of your colleagues will be willing to share helpful insights; others may set you up for a fall. Be careful. If a person talks negatively about others, don't get involved. Do not comment. Something that you innocently say will more than likely get back to the person and will make you appear to be the culprit. You can't be sure, so don't take a chance. Keep in mind; the person who talks about others will soon get around to talking about you. It is good practice restraint. Refrain from contributing to this negative grapevine. Never say things you don't want heard because they always seem to get repeated. People will tell you things in confidence. If you make the mistake of telling others what was told to you, you may cause serious relation problems for yourself and others. Never say anything you don't want repeated, and never repeat what is told to you in confidence.

The grapevine is not always negative according to McKay. She declares that gossip can have its place in the workplace and it can be beneficial. In many workplaces, the office grapevine is the only means of transmitting important news. She suggests that you make the grapevine work for you. Begin by taking a critical look at what you hear. Confirm that it is true before you act on it. If you contribute the grapevine, keep in mind that what you say may get distorted. You can use the grapevine to your advantage. If you had a great success at work or worked hard on a project, this is information you want to share. You never know whom it will reach.

RoAne's view of office politics supports the positive side. She tells us that office politics have a dramatic effect on your organization and on your personal career. She indicates that you must be able to separate your skills as a professional from that needed to compete politically. Political skill requires awareness of how the organization operates and who operates it, as well as the unwritten and written rules. The lack of political savvy in the workplace has its disadvantages. You may be perceived as:

- Lacking a career management skill
- Being unpromotable
- Being a loner, rather than a team player
- Lacking logic, practicality, savvy, and know-how
- Being untrustworthy of confidences and critical information

The following strategies can be used to increase your political know-how:

- Observe your colleagues, subordinates, and supervisors – With whom do they interact and socialize?
- Read the body language of colleagues when names and assignments are mentioned
- Listen to conversations in the staff room and in other unofficial places such as the washroom

While this type of informal listening may be considered as eavesdropping and perceived as negative, it provides certain information that you may not get otherwise. It may allow you to learn of birthdays, anniversaries, the loss of a loved one by a colleague, and other such information, and to take the appropriate steps to acknowledge these events.

RoAne also concludes that the office grapevine has received a tremendous amount of bad press, some of which is not deserved. She believes that if used properly, it can provide a great deal of useful information and be a powerful career aid. She suggests that those who consider informal communication to be gossip consider the following:

- Information is not necessarily personal gossip, 80 percent of it is probably business-related office politics.
- Gossip can be an intentional leak by top management of information you should know.
- Conveying a superior attitude about the grapevine could eliminate your source of information.
- Smart people manage their careers. Cultivating sources of information make sense.

If you are not already experienced at cultivating the grapevine, RoAne offers the following tips.

- Determine who has access to relevant, powerful sources of information.
- Trade information when it's required.
- Don't fan the flame of gossip with your opinion.
- Observe colleagues and those with whom they interact and socialize.
- Buy lunch for those who are prime grapevine sources.
- Recognize that members of professional associations may have information about the organization.
- The grapevine now has its own web – become a web savvy networker.
- Don't e-mail that which may return to haunt you.

Sharing Personal Business

Sharing personal business with colleagues can be a sticky situation. It's kind of hard not to because you spend most of your time with them. However, there are several reasons for not sharing personal information with your colleagues. Keeping a secret can be a burden and you may not want to burden your colleagues in this way. Then, there is the issue of trust, or lack of trust may be more accurate. You cannot always trust your colleagues to keep your secret. Some people assume there's nothing wrong with telling others whatever you told them and innocently share the information with others. Then, there are those who will think nothing of talking about you and will maliciously spread information with the express intention of causing you harm. By the time you find out you've shared your information with the wrong person it's usually too late.

There are many personal things that you can share with colleagues, but the more private and intimate personal and family issues are not to be shared. You should want to maintain some level of personal privacy in the workplace. This also means that you afford your colleagues the same privacy by refraining from prying into their personal business. When you share too much personal information, especially information that shows your weaknesses, you may compromise your professional position. In this case a lack of privacy can very well become problematic. Colleagues and subordinates may perceive you differently and, in turn, respond to you differently. Revealing too much about yourself may give people the wrong impression or rather the impression you don't want them to have. Sharing too much personal information can have a negative impact on productivity and can emotionally charge the work environment. Ultimately, the decision about how much to share or not to share is yours. And the consequences are also yours.

Office Romance

Office romance is a controversial topic. Some consider it be disastrous, while others contend that it may not be such a bad thing. Many sources report that interoffice dating can be risky for your love life and for your career. On the other hand, an increasing number of sources say that it can be an asset and argue that working with your lover is the ultimate form of work/life balance. In either case, whether it is an asset or a liability will depend on the maturity and values of the individuals involved and how the relationship turns out.

There is general agreement that office romance has negative aspects and can possibly be a liability for the individuals involved and for the organization. Common side effects of office romance include: feelings of awkwardness and discomfort, harboring of negative feelings toward each other, and emotional distress. At the extreme, there can be even more serious negative repercussions resulting in violence in the workplace.
Office romance can also create awkward situations among colleagues. Claims of favoritism may surface and participants can become the subject of contagious gossip that can hurt professional credibility and damage careers. If lovers are caught doing something inappropriate at the workplace or if one decides to sue the other for sexual harassment (see Chapter 10), one or both can begin the search for a new job.

Office romance gone badly can be as hard or even harder on the organization. The potential for sexual harassment charges and revenge-motivated complaints are multiplied and organizations are worried about liability. Some organizations are now using contracts to counter sexual harassment charges and other office romance related problems. The contract is called a "consensual relationship agreement." It is signed by the couple and specifies that the relationship is mutually agreeable, consensual, and unrelated to the organization; that they are aware of and know how to apply the organizations policy against sexual harassment; and that they agree to settle any relationship dispute through binding arbitration, not a lawsuit.

If you make the decision to become involved in an office romance, know what you are getting into. It is recommended by the *i*Village Job Resource Center that you adhere to the following rules.

- **Know your organizations policy.**

  Dating colleagues is not illegal; however, some organizations have policies against it. Even though your organization cannot legally hold a relationship against you, you can assume that it is not acceptable. There is one corporate rule that is wise to follow: if the person you want to date is a supervisor or a subordinate, it is best to forgo the relationship.

- **Establish ground rules from the start.**

  Discuss what your expectations of each other are. Decide whom you will tell about your relationship. Decide how you will interact at work. And even though it may be easier said than done, agree that you will be friends in the event that you breakup.

- **Be aware of perceptions.**

  Be aware that office romance can affect others perceptions of your professional identity. You might well be perceived as demonstrating inappropriate use of power or even creating a hostile environment.

- **How will it affect your job?**

  New relationships can be a big distraction. Having your partner in the office with you can make things more complicated and even more distracting. Be certain that your relation does not negatively affect your production.

- **Be discreet.**

  It is not necessary to broadcast your relationship to everyone in the office. Keep your business to yourself. Refrain from displaying intimacies in the workplace.

Be Yourself

It is important for you to be yourself. Starting a new job will require you to adjust to a new situation. You may be nervous and have some feelings of inadequacy. It's natural and most people have the same reactions. Your colleagues will recognize that you are a fake and will not trust you. Trying to be something that you're not can be exhausting. Spend you energy learning and performing your job. You have gotten this far by being yourself; you can succeed by being yourself.

DEVELOP AN EXIT PLAN

In today's world of work, careers are short-term. Don't take your job for granted. On any given day and for any number of reasons, your job could end. On the other hand, you may think of your job as a stepping-stone in the process of building your career. Develop an exit plan that will include how long you will stay in the job, when you will leave, and what you want to leave with. What skills do you want to acquire? What types of contacts do you want to have? What kind of new knowledge do you want to have? In addition, keep a file documenting all the successes that you have had. Your file will be useful if you leave or if you stay. This type plan will help you prepare for both the expected and the unexpected. Remember where you are headed and make sure your career keeps going in that direction.

SUMMARY

The first year of your career is a unique and critical period. Research shows that your success with the organization, future salary, career satisfaction, and other aspects of career are affected by your approach to the first year. It is important to enter the organization with the appropriate expectations and attitudes.

Entering the organization for the first time, you must learn the culture, earn respect and credibility, and establish yourself. You learn the culture by observing the dynamics of the workplace. You earn respect and credibility by giving respect and "paying your dues." You establish yourself by demonstrating your maturity and professionalism. Professionalism has three dimensions: professional behavior, lifelong learning, and involvement in the profession. Professional behavior indicates a commitment to professional practice and ethical standards. Lifelong learning signifies a commitment to professional growth. Involvement indicates participation in the profession on a broader scale. Each dimension is essential in your development as a professional and contributes to success in your career.

If you work diligently, professionally and courteously, your colleagues will come forward with respect, warmth, and acceptance. The key to a successful success first year is to be conservative in your behavior and your attitudes and focus on understanding who and what you are dealing with.

REFLECTIONS

1. Reflect on yourself as a beginning professional. Think of some ways in which you can successfully enter a new organization?

2. Reflect on your current or past job experiences. Identify times when you participated in office dynamics. Evaluate the situations and determine what could have been done to minimize or eliminate the situation. Use Laboratory 9.2 for your response.

WEB SITES

www.cdm.uwaterloo.ca
Career Development eManual

http://careerplanning.about.com
Career planning and job hunting

www.fastcompany.com/career/salary.html
Research salaries

www.careerbuilder.com
Careers Network

www.jobweb.com
Jobweb

BIBLIOGRAPHY

Alesko, M. (2002). Office Politics. *Today's Careers*. www.today's-careers.com.

Accountemps. (1998). Surviving Office Politics. *Talent Scout*. April 16, 1998. www.careerplanning.about.com/library/weekly/aa041998.htm.

Buley, J. (2000). What is a Professional? It Starts Now, Not When You Graduate. http://com.pp.asu.edu/aca/Professional.html.

Dukass, K. (2002). Don't expect a honeymoon when starting a new job. *USA Today Careers Network*.

Harr, J. and Hess, K. (2005). *Seeking Employment in Careers in Criminal Justice and Related Fields: From Internships to Professionalism,* 5th ed. Belmont, CA: Thomson Wadsworth.

Holton, E. (1998). *The Ultimate New Employee Survival Guide*. Princeton, New Jersey. Peterson's.

IVillage Resource Center. (2002). Workplace Romance: 5 Smart Dating Tips. www.ivillage.com/work/job/succeed/articles/0,10109,187833_98023,00.html.

McKay, D. (2002). Does Gossip Have a Place at Work? www.careerplanning.about.com.

Parkay F. and Stanford, B. (2001). *Becoming a Teacher*, 5th ed. Boston, MA: Allyn and Bacon.

RoAne, S. (2002). Office Politics: A You a Naysayer? www.susanroane.com/articles/offpols.html.

LABORATORY ACTIVITY 9.1

NAME _____ DATE _____

COURSE _____ SECTION _____

Identify a career that you would consider entering. Interview a supervisor from the organization
to determine some of the mistakes that new employees make and what can be done to minimize these
mistakes. Discuss the results of your research with the class.

LABORATORY ACTIVITY 9.2

NAME _____ DATE _____

COURSE _____ SECTION _____

Review the "Office Dynamics" section of the chapter. Reflect on your current or past job experiences. Identify examples of occurrences of the dynamics on your job. In small groups, discuss the effect that the dynamics had on the working environment and what could have been done to minimize or eliminate the situation. Share the results of your discussion with the class.

CHAPTER 10

LEGAL ISSUES

"Experience is not what happens to you, it is what you do with what happens to you."
Aldous Huxley

KEY CONCEPTS

1. It is illegal to discriminate against employees because of their age, ethnicity, religion, gender, disability, sexual orientation, or national origin.
2. There is no federal law that specifically outlaws workplace discrimination on the basis of sexual orientation in the private sector.
3. Sexual harassment is any unwelcome sexual advance or conduct on the job that creates an intimidating, hostile or offensive working environment
4. There are legal and illegal questions during a job interview.
5. Learning how to communicate among cultures is necessary no matter what type of career you choose.

INTRODUCTION

Society is demanding so much more from its employers today than it has in the past. It is necessary to be knowledgeable and to understand the rights and legal duties one has in the workplace. Every employer/employee has the potential to be involved in a lawsuit; no one is immune. The first step in avoiding litigation and protecting your rights is to take a positive approach and do what is best for you and your organization.

Knowledge, preparation, and prevention are the most important factors in protecting oneself against a potential lawsuit and wrong doing. To protect yourself, you must be knowledgeable about legal guidelines for school personnel (teacher and administrators) and/or employee/employer rights and responsibilities both generally and in your chosen career field. Litigation has caused programs to be suspended, organizations and facilities to be closed, equipment to be banned and careers to be placed on hold until legal issues are settled. Lawsuits can provoke chaos on personnel, programs, and the reputation of an organization. Policies and procedures underlying legal actions are similar, but certain procedures and regulations may vary from state to state. Educate yourself on the laws relative to discrimination and harassment. Become knowledgeable of what the laws are, how they are proven in court, and what your responsibilities are as an employee. Issues of concern include discrimination and harassment, family and medical leave, health and safety, workplace diversity, and job interview questions.

DISCRIMINATION AND HARASSMENT ISSUES

It is difficult enough to get and to keep a job in today's society. When an employer mistreats you it is even more challenging. The federal and state governments have provided some legal protection of equal treatment in the workplace for discrimination and harassment issues that include: age, ethnicity, religion, gender, disability, sexual orientation, and national origin. Sexual harassment will be discussed as an independent issue.

Age

State and federal laws protect employees from discrimination on the basis of their age. The Federal Age Discrimination in Employment Act (ADEA) is the federal law that prohibits employers from discriminating against employees and applicants who are 40 years of age or older on the basis of their age.

The ADEA prohibits discrimination in all phases of the employment relationship, except benefits and early retirement, which are addressed by a different law. ADEA applies to all private employers that have 20 or more employees. ADEA applies to the federal government, but not to the state government.

The ADEA prohibit discrimination against older workers in favor of those who are younger than 40 but also prohibits discrimination among older workers. For example, an employer cannot hire a 33-year-old over a 53-year-old simply because of age.

Many state laws mirror the federal law and only protect people older than 40. Other laws are broader and protect workers of all ages. State laws tend to include employers with fewer than 20 employees. Contact your state labor department and your state fair employment office for more information about age discrimination. See websites located at the end of this chapter.

Ethnicity

Federal law and the laws of the 50 states prohibit discrimination and harassment in employment based on ethnicity. It is illegal to treat an employee or applicant differently because of his or her ethnicity or color in regard to all phases of the employment relationship, including: help-wanted ads, interviews, pre-employment testing, hiring, job assignments, shift assignments, promotions, compensation, benefits, job training, layoffs or termination. This prohibition also includes discrimination based on stereotypes or assumptions about people of a certain ethnicity. For example, if you think people of a certain ethnicity or lazy or are prone to violence.

These laws also prohibit harassment based on certain ethnic characteristics such as skin color, hair texture or other physical features. Harassment occurs any time people are forced to endure a work environment that is hostile, intimidating, or offensive to them because of their ethnicity or color. Harassing acts can include:

- Ethnic slurs/jokes
- Offensive remarks or comments based on ethnicity
- Drawings or pictures that depict people of a certain ethnicity in an unfavorable light
- Threats
- Intimidation
- Hostile demeanor, or
- Physical violence

These laws also prohibit employers from retaliating against people who complain or who assert their rights under these laws. For example, you cannot fire someone for complaining about ethnic discrimination. Refer to the website of the U.S. Equal Employment Opportunity Commission for more information about ethnicity discrimination laws.

Religion

Title VII of the Civil Rights Act and most state laws prohibit employers from discriminating on the basis of religious beliefs. Employers are generally required to accommodate employees who articulate a need to express their religious beliefs and practices in the workplace.

Employers have flexibility in how they accommodate employees. An employer is not required to accept whatever accommodation the employee suggests, or to spare the employee all expenses in making the accommodation. For example, the employer may give the day off for religious observation, but without pay. In addition, employers are not required to make accommodations that would cause them undue hardship. An accommodation that would require more than minimal cost to the employer, considering its size and resources, would be considered an undue hardship. Courts make different decisions about what is an undue burden for employers. Therefore, it would be best for both the employer and employee to work together to reach a mutually acceptable accommodation and keep the issue out of court.

Gender

Many legal issues are centered on gender. When gender and gender relations are discussed, the topics usually focus on issues related to fairness and equity. Fairness and equity issues revolve around topics such as pregnancy, equal pay for equal work, and office romance.

Pregnancy

The Pregnancy Discrimination Act is an amendment to Title VII of the Civil Rights Act of 1964. Discrimination on the basis of pregnancy, childbirth or related medical conditions constitutes unlawful sex discrimination under Title VII. Women affected by pregnancy or related conditions must be treated in the same manner as other applicants or employees with similar abilities or limitations.

An employer cannot refuse to hire a woman because of her pregnancy related condition as long as she is able to perform the major functions of her job. An employer cannot refuses to hire her because of its prejudices against pregnant workers or the prejudices of co-workers, clients or customers.

If an employer requires its employees to submit a doctor's statement concerning their inability to work before granting leave or paying sick benefits, the employer may require employees affected by pregnancy related conditions to submit such statements.

If an employee is temporarily unable to perform her job due to pregnancy, the employer must treat her the same as any other temporarily disabled employee: for example, by providing modified tasks, alternative assignments, disability leave or leave without pay.

Pregnant employees must be permitted to work as long as they are able to perform their job. If an employee has been absent from work as a result of a pregnancy related condition and recovers, her employer may not require her to remain on leave until the baby's birth. An employer may or may not have a rule which prohibits an employee from returning to work for a predetermined length of time after childbirth. Employers must hold open a job for a pregnancy related absences the same length of time jobs are held open for employees on sick or disability leave.

Any health insurance provided by an employer must cover expenses for pregnancy related conditions on the same basis as costs for other medical conditions. Health insurance arising from abortion is not required, except where the life of the mother is endangered.

Pregnancy related benefits cannot be limited to married employees. If an employer provides any benefits to workers on leave, the employer must provide the same benefits for those on leave for pregnancy related condition. Employees with pregnancy related disabilities must be treated the same as other temporarily disable employees for accrual and crediting of seniority, vacation calculation, pay increases and temporary disability benefits.

Equal Pay for Equal Work

The Equal Pay Act, a federal law passed in 1963 as an amendment to the Fair Labor Standards Act, requires employers to pay all employees equally for equal work, regardless of their gender. Equal Pay Act covers professional employees, executives and managers, and administrators and teachers in elementary and secondary schools. Even though the Act protects both women and men from gender discrimination in pay rates, it was passed to help rectify the problems faced by women workers because of sex discrimination in employment. In practice, this law has almost always been applied to situations where women are being paid less than men for doing similar jobs.

Since 1980, women's earning was only 60 percent of men's. The 2000 figure has women earning about 75 percent as much as working men. The law's biggest weakness is that it applies only when men and women are doing the same work. Since women have historically been banned from many types of work and had only limited entrée to managerial positions, the Equal Pay Act in reality affects very few women.

To successfully raise a claim under the Equal Pay Act, you must show that the two employees, both male and female are:

- Working in the same place
- Doing equal work
- Receiving unequal pay

Jobs do not have to be identical for the courts to consider them equal. Courts have ruled that two jobs are equal for the purposes of the Equal Pay Act when both require equal levels of skill, effort and responsibility and are performed under similar conditions. Job titles, classifications and descriptions may or may not weigh into the determination.

According to a recent nationwide survey by the AFL-CIO, money is foremost in the minds of America's working women. Asked to cite their top workplace concerns, about 94 percent of the women polled rated equal pay for equal work, 33 percent noted childcare, 78 percent cited sexual harassment, and 72 percent mentioned downsizing. According to the Institute for Women's Policy Research, women earn $24,000 annually – much less than men's $32,000 yearly average. If these figures hold, today's 25 year-old woman who puts in 40 years of work before retiring will earn about a half million fewer dollars than a male worker at the same age and stage.

Office Romance

Office romance may or may not be of concern. It depends on the individuals involved. In some situations it may work, while in another situation it could interfere with one or both individuals in their productivity on the job. In essence, there is no federal law protecting couples, but there are laws about discrimination –treating people differently because of gender or ethnicity. If you exclude one person in a relationship by firing, demoting or moving them, it is discrimination. See Chapter 10 for more information on Office Romance.

Disability

Since its passage in 1990, the Americans With Disabilities Act (ADA) makes it illegal to discriminate against disabled individuals in employment, public accommodations, public services, and telecommunications. According to the ADA, "an individual is considered to have a disability if s/he has a physical or mental impairment that substantially limits one or more major life activities, has a record of such an impairment, or is regarded as having such an impairment." Title I of the ADA covers employment and, since 1994, requires that employers of more than 15 people must make reasonable accommodations that allow a qualified job applicant with a disability to complete the application process or a disabled employee to carry out the duties of his or her job.

It is illegal to require a job candidate to take a medical examination prior to a job offer being made, however the employer may require the candidate to demonstrate the ability to perform the job in question. It is up to the job candidate to decide when and if to disclose a disability that is considered invisible, a chronic illness that shows no visual symptoms, or a psychiatric disorder. The National Alliance for the Mentally Ill has published the *Americans With Disabilities: Helpline Fact Sheet*, which discusses the Americans With Disabilities Act as it applies to those with a mental impairment. Employers must make reasonable accommodations for those who are mentally ill, just as they must for those with physical disabilities. The impact on the workplace will be substantial, according to *Accommodating Employees: Impact of Newly Released Guidelines For Mentally Ill,* since "one out of four people in the workplace need mental health services."

Individuals who suffer from a serious illness may take job protected leave under The Family and Medical Leave Act of 1993 (FMLA), a federal law. *The Family and Medical Leave Act Q & A* is a comprehensive reference tool that answers questions about the FMLA.

Sexual Orientation

A growing number of laws prohibit discrimination against gay and lesbian employees. On the job discrimination is often present in the form of homophobic comments and jokes, messages and pictures on bulletin boards, e-mail pictures and jokes, and lectures about upholding the organization's image. Promotions are often denied and jobs are even lost because of sexual orientation. Employers are finding that they are responsible for providing a workplace free of discrimination and harassment.

According to the National Gay and Lesbian Taskforce, approximately 62 percent of the gay and lesbian populations have no legislative protection from workplace discrimination based on sexual orientation, particularly in the private sector. Courts are split on whether there is legal protection for workers who do not openly identify themselves as gay but who are discriminated against because the employer believes they are gay.

Women, minorities, people older than 40 and people with disabilities now enjoy an umbrella of state and federal protections from discrimination in the workplace. Gays and lesbians have, for the most part, been left out especially at the national level. However, federal government workers are currently protected from such discrimination. Seven states have passed legislation prohibiting sexual orientation discrimination in public jobs and eleven states have laws prohibiting sexual orientation discrimination in both private and public jobs. If your state does not have a law for protection in the workplace, city and county ordinances may offer protection. There is no federal law that specifically outlaws workplace discrimination on the basis of sexual orientation in the private sector Many companies have adopted their own policies prohibiting such discrimination.

If you are gay or lesbian and you need assistance you can visit the Lambda Legal Defense and Education Fund website or contact the Lambda office in your region. A volunteer will assist you or refer you to a volunteer attorney. Information about gay and lesbian workplace rights can be provided from the National Gay and Lesbian Task Force.

National Origin

Title VII of the Civil Rights Act of 1964 protects individuals against employment discrimination on the basis of race, color, religion and sex as well as national origin. It is unlawful to discriminate against any employee or applicant because of the individual's national origin. No one can be denied equal employment opportunity because of birthplace, ancestry, culture, or linguistic characteristics common to a specific ethnic group. Equal employment opportunity cannot be denied because of marriage or association with persons of a national origin group; membership or association with specific ethnic promotion groups; attendance or participation in schools, churches, temples or mosques generally associated with a national origin group; or a surname associated with a national origin group.

SEXUAL HARASSMENT

It is the employers' legal obligation to maintain a workplace that is free of sexual harassment. Sexual harassment in the workplace contributes to poor employee morale, low productivity and lawsuits. Sexual harassment is any unwelcome sexual advance or conduct on the job that creates an intimidating, hostile or offensive working environment. In reality, both men and women are subject to sexual harassment. Sexually harassing behavior ranges from offensive or belittling jokes, offensive pornography, e-mails, bulletin or announcement boards with pictures or jokes, implied and explicit sexual overtures, and outright sexual assault.

The same laws that prohibit gender discrimination prohibit sexual harassment. Title VII of the Civil Rights Act in federal Anti-Discrimination Laws is the specific federal law that prohibits sexual harassment. Each state has its own anti-sexual harassment law. In 1986, the U.S. Supreme Court first ruled that sexual harassment was a form of job discrimination, thus becoming illegal. To find out the law in your state, call 800-669-4000 and ask for the federal EEOC office nearest you. See websites located at the end of this chapter.

Preventive Strategies for the Employer

- Clearly say you want the offensive behavior to stop. Some experts say up to 90 percentage of the time this works.

- Document incidents by keeping a diary or journal to later prove that the harassment continued after you confronted the harasser.

- If the harasser ignored your oral requests to stop or you are uncomfortable talking to the harasser face to face, write a succinct letter demanding an end to the behavior and save a copy.

- If your oral requests do not end the harassment, escalate your complaint within the organization. Talk to your supervisor and/or manager about what is going on. Keep the lines of communication open.

- Check your company's handbook, personnel policies or manual. If there is not a policy, ask someone in the human resources or personnel department how to make a sexual harassment complaint. If you do not use the company's internal complaint procedure to make the company aware of the problem, you cannot later hold the company liable in a lawsuit for the harassment.

- Place your company on notice of the harassment even if the organization does not have a formal complaint procedure. You can make a complaint to the human resources department, inform your supervisor of the problem or send a letter to an organization administrator or executive.

- Collect detailed evidence about the specifics of your harassment. Save offensive letters, photographs, cards, notes or e-mails you receive. Make copies or confiscate jokes, pin-ups or cartoons posted on boards or walls. An anonymous, obnoxious photo or joke posted on a bulletin board is not anyone else's personal property, so feel free to take it down and keep it as evidence. Keep copies of e-mails, photograph the workplace wall, note the dates the offensive material was posted and whether there was hostile reaction when you took it down or asked another person to do so.

- Keep a detailed journal Write down the specifics of everything that feels like harassment. Include the name of everyone involved, what happened, where and when it took place. If anyone else said or heard the harassment, note that as well. Be as specific as possible about what was said and done and how it affected you, your health or job performance.

- Make copies of your periodic written evaluation of your work. Ask for a copy of your entire personnel file, before you inform them that you are considering taking action against a harassing co-worker. Your records will be persuasive evidence if your evaluation has been good but after you complain, your employer retaliates by trying to transfer or fire you, claiming poor job performance.

- If the investigation and settlement attempts fail to produce satisfactory results, file a civil lawsuit for damages under the federal Civil Rights Act or under a state fair employment practices statute. You may have to first file a claim with a government agency. The EEOC or state agency may decide to prosecute your case on its own, but that happens only occasionally. At some point the agency will issue you a document referred to as a "right-to-sue" letter that allows you to take your case to court.

- Be cooperative but cautious when dealing with government agencies. When the employee makes a complaint with a government agency (either the Federal Equal Employment Opportunity Commission (EEOC) or an equivalent state agency), that agency may ask you to provide certain documents, to give your opinion and to explain any efforts you made to deal the complaint. Provide the agency with the materials requested, but remember that the agency is gathering evidence that could be used against you later. This may be the best time to hire a lawyer to advise you.

Prevention Strategies for Employer

There are several strategies that can be used by employers to reduce the risk of sexual harassment occurring in the workplace. Employers can:

- Adopt a clear sexual harassment policy. Place this policy in the employee handbook. The policy should define sexual harassment, state in no uncertain terms that it will not tolerated, state that any wrongdoers will disciplined or fired, set out a clear procedure for filing complaints, state that will investigate fully any complaint that you receive and that you will not tolerate retaliation against anyone who complains about sexual harassment.

- Train employees. At least once a year, conduct training sessions for employees. Educate them about sexual harassment policies and procedures.

- Train supervisors and managers. At least once a year conduct training sessions for supervisors and manager that are separate from the employee sessions. Educate them about sexual harassment and provide detailed instruction on how to deal with complaints.

- Monitor the workplace. Get out among the employees periodically. Talk to them about the work environment. Ask for their opinions and perceptions.

- Take all complaints seriously. Act immediately to investigate a complaint. If the complaint is valid, the response should be swift and effective.

Men can sexually harass women, and women can sexually harass men. Whether sexual harassment of gays and lesbians is illegal is an open question now and the subject of debate. The U.S. Supreme Court has never addressed the issue, and lower federal courts and state courts have various opinions about the issue.

When filing an action for sexual harassment, you will most likely need to hire a lawyer for help. For more information about sexual harassment contact the 9 to 5 National Association of Working Women, 800-522-0925 (Hotline). See websites located at the end of this chapter.

FAMILY AND MEDICAL LEAVE ACT (FMLA)

President Bill Clinton signed FMLA into law in 1993. It requires certain employers to give their workers up to 12 weeks off per year to care for a seriously ill family member, recuperate from their own serious illness or take care of a newborn or newly adopted child. Employers must allow employees to take paid time off (such as vacation and sick time), provide employees with continued health insurance while on leave during FMLA leave under certain circumstances, and reinstate an employee to the position s/he held before taking leave. Employers can refuse to reinstate certain highly paid employees if they are among the 10 percent of most highly paid salaried workforce and reinstating would cause "substantial and grievous economic injury" to the company.

An employee is entitled to FMLA leave when these conditions are met:

- Number of employees. The employer has 50 or more employees who work within a 75-mile radius. All employees on the payroll, including part-time workers and workers out on leave, count toward the total.

- Length of time employed. The employee has worked for the employer for at least 12 months.

- Hours worked. The employee has worked at least 1,250 hours (about 25 hours a week) during the 12 months immediately preceding the leave.

HEALTH AND SAFETY

The federal law covering threats to workplace safety is the Occupational Safety and Health Act of 1970 (OSHA). OSHA requires employers to provide a workplace that is free of dangers that could physically harm employees.

This law requires that employers protect employees from "recognized hazards" in the workplace. It does not specify or limit the types of dangers covered. It includes those hazards likely to cause death or serious physical injury.

Approximately half of the states have their own OSHA laws and most protections are similar to the federal law. State laws usually concentrate on protecting workers who complain about safety violations from being demoted or fired. Some states, for example, Texas has instituted a 24-hour hotline to receive complaints and prohibits employers from discriminating against those who call in.

The first step to take if you feel that your workplace is unsafe is to make your supervisor aware of the danger. Follow up with written communication if your supervisor does not take prompt action. If you are still unsuccessful, contact a higher-level administrator/executive to correct the safety hazard. If all else fails, file a complaint at the nearest OSHA office. The U.S. Labor Department in the federal government section of your local telephone directory can provide additional assistance on this issue.

ILLEGAL REASONS FOR FIRING EMPLOYEES

Both state and federal law prohibits employers from using certain reasons to fire an employee. These prohibitions apply regardless of whether the employee has a contract for employment or not. These reasons include:

Discrimination

Federal law makes it illegal for most employers to fire an employee on the basis of age, ethnicity, religion, gender, disability, sexual orientation, or national origin. Many state laws are broader than federal laws. Additional prohibitions such as sexual orientation or marital status are included.

Retaliation

It is illegal for employers to fire employees for asserting their rights under the state and federal anti-discrimination laws described previously.

Lie Detector Test

The federal Employee Polygraph Protection Act prohibits most employers from terminating employees for refusing to take a lie detector test. Many state laws also concur with federal law.

Alien Status

The federal Immigration Reform and Control Act (IRCA) prohibit most employers from using an employee's alien status as a reason for terminating that employee so long as that employee is legally eligible to work in the United States.

OSHA Violation Complaint

The federal Occupational Safety and Health Act (OSHA) makes it illegal for employers to fire employees for complaining that work conditions fall short of complying with state or federal health and safety rules.

Violations of Public Policy

Most states prohibit employers from firing an employee in violation of public policy, that is, for reasons that most people would find morally or ethically wrong. The law will vary from state to state, while some states may include violations that other states do not. Public Policy violations include terminating an employee for:

- Refusing to commit an illegal act such as refusing to falsify insurance claims

- Complaining about illegal practices such as failure to pay minimum wage

- Exercising a legal right such as voting or other political activity.

GUIDELINES FOR HANDLING DISCRIMINATION AND HARASSMENT COMPLAINTS

Employee's complaints can lead to workplace tension, government investigations and costly long-term legal battles. When a complaint is mishandled, even unintentionally, an employer may unwittingly put him/herself and the organization in long-term litigation that can be harmful to all involved. When the employer takes the complaint seriously and follows a careful and well thought out strategy for dealing with it, the employer can reduce the likelihood of a lawsuit and even improve employee relations in the process. The employer should:

- **Be open-minded**

  Each complaint received should be investigated. Drawing conclusions should be avoided until the investigation is completed. Many employers fail to investigate complaints assuming that these complaints cannot be true. This is a costly mistake that could lead to litigation.

- **Treat the complainer with compassion and respect**

  Often employees find it difficult to complain about situations at work. They feel afraid and vulnerable. This can have an impact on the quality of their work and lead them to seek outside assistance from lawyers. Employers should be understanding when an employee comes in with concerns about problems in the workplace. When employees feel that their complaints are taken seriously and that supervisors will not become angry with them for complaining they are less likely to take complaints to a government agency or to lawyers.

- **Place no blame on the complainer**

  Employers may be tempted to become angry with the complainer for having to deal with these situations. Remember that the complaining employee is the victim and not the cause of the problem. Becoming angry may lead to claims of illegal retaliation, damaging morale and lowering productivity.

- **Refrain from retaliation**

  It is against the law to punish someone for complaining about discrimination or harassment. Subtle forms of retaliation may include changing the work area or job responsibilities, isolating the complainer by leaving her/him out of meetings or other office functions, or changing working hours.

- **Follow the procedures**

  Check the employee handbook or other documented policies relating to the charges and follow these policies.

- **Interview the people involved**

  Interview the complainer to find out exactly what the concerns are. Get details on what was said or done, when, where, and who else was there. Take notes of interviews. Talk to any employees who are being accused of discrimination or harassment and get details from them as well.

- **Look for corroboration or contradiction**

  Discrimination complaints often offer the classic example of "he said/she said." Interview any witnesses who may have seen or heard any problematic conduct. Gather any relevant documents such as schedules, attendance records, or other information. For example: It is hard to argue with an email that contains ethnic slurs or sexual innuendo.

- **Keep it confidential**

  A discrimination complaint can upset a workplace. Employees will likely side with either the complaining employee or the accused employee. The rumor mill will start working overtime. If too many details about the complaint are disclosed charges of damaging the reputation of the alleged victim or alleged harasser may arise and result in a defamation lawsuit. Insisting on confidentiality and practicing it throughout the investigation should avoid these problems.

- **Document it**

  Take notes during interviews. Before the interview is over, the interviewer should review notes with the interviewee to make sure the information is correct. Keep a journal of the investigation. Write down the steps taken to get at the truth, including dates and places of interviews conducted. Write down the names of all documents reviewed. Document any action taken against the accused or the reasons for deciding not to take action. This information will be useful later if any claim that the complaint was ignored or conducted unfairly or improperly arise.

- **Cooperate with government agencies**

  Be cooperative, but cautious when dealing with government agencies. When the employee makes a complaint with a government agency (either the Federal Equal Employment Opportunity Commission (EEOC) or an equivalent state agency), employers answer questions and supply written documents as requested.

- **Consider hiring an experienced investigator**

  Many law firms and private consulting agencies will investigate workplace complaints for a fee. An external investigator may hired if more than one employee complains of harassment, the accused is a high-ranking official in your organization (principal, CEO, superintendent), the accused has publicized the complaint in the workplace or in the media, if the accusations are extreme (allegations of assault, or rape) or if the workplace investigator is too personally involved to a make a fair, objective decision.

- **Take appropriate action**

  Once the information is gathered decisions must be made. If it is concluded that some form of discrimination or harassment occurred, disciplining the guilty person should occur quickly and appropriately. Termination may be warranted for more egregious kinds of discrimination and harassment, such as stalking, threats, or repeated and unwanted physical contact. Lesser discipline, such as a warning or counseling might be in order if the harassment arises out of a misunderstanding or less serious situations.

WORKPLACE DIVERSITY

Definitions of workplace diversity are still evolving and there continues to be different definitions of diversity. More women, more ethnic minorities, and more immigrants are entering the work force. Thus, the workplace is increasingly multicultural. Some feel that workplace diversity means an office environment that includes both full- and part-time staff. To some, it means being surrounded by people of other cultures, ethnicities, nationalities, sexual orientations, and faiths. To others it means abiding by the equal employment opportunity laws. While others have little or no understanding of the concept.

"Workplace diversity," unlike "equal opportunity," and "affirmative action" is not a legal term, nor does it necessarily refer to discriminatory hiring practices. It describes a much broader effort by employers to maintain a workforce that more accurately represents the complexity of today's society.

As industries grow more dependent on a global marketplace including new clients and employees, they are realizing that diversity policies help them capture a larger market share, and identify previously hidden opportunities for growth. The first step in defining diversity is to understand how "workplace diversity" differs from "equal employment opportunity" and "affirmative action programs."

Equal Employment Opportunity (EEO)

EEO refers to five specific federal laws that prohibit discrimination on the basis of ethnicity, color, religion, gender, national origin, physical handicap, or mental handicap. The Federal Equal Employment Opportunity Commission enforces these laws.

Title VII of the Civil Rights Act of 1964

Title VII prohibits employment discrimination because of race, color, sex, national origin, and religion. It also prohibits retaliation for opposing discrimination, filing a complaint, or participating in a related proceeding.

Age Discrimination in Employment Act of 1967 (ADEA)

ADEA prohibits employment discrimination because of age against persons age 40 and older. It also prohibits retaliation for opposing age discrimination, filing a complaint, or participating in a related proceeding. This law was amended by the Older Workers Benefit Protection Act, which sets minimum criteria that must be satisfied before a waiver of any ADEA right is considered a "knowing and voluntary" waiver.

Americans With Disabilities Act of 1990, Titles I and V

This federal law prohibits employment discrimination because of mental and physical disabilities that substantially limit a major life activity; or having a record of a disability; or being regarded as having a disability. It requires reasonable accommodation of mental and physical disabilities.

Civil Rights Act of 1991

The Civil Rights Act provides for the recovery of compensatory and punitive damages in actions under Title VII and the Americans With Disabilities Act, and addresses other aspects of discrimination law, including disparate impact claims, mixed motive cases, seniority systems, coverage of U. S. citizens employed abroad by American corporations, and expert witness fees.

Equal Pay Act of 1963

This law prohibits wage differentials based on sex for jobs that require equal skill, effort, and responsibility, and are performed under similar working conditions in the same establishment ("equal pay for equal work").

Affirmative Action

"Affirmative action" refers to specific plans employers themselves write as guidelines for actively seeking a more diverse workforce. These plans typically address how to hire more people from traditionally underrepresented groups, and how best to replace past and present discriminatory practices with appropriate remedies. Four common types of affirmative action that employers use involve:

- Aggressive recruiting practices to expand the pool of potential candidates
- Updating hiring tools and guidelines to ensure relevance to job performance
- Expanding the way merit, talent, and performance are measured
- Setting up goals and timetables for recruitment and retention.

California, Florida and some other states are challenging the constitutionality of affirmative action programs. Opponents say such programs provide certain groups with an unfair advantage, or force employers to hire less-qualified candidates simply to fill quotas. Because of the controversy, many employers shy away from discussions of "equal opportunity" and "affirmative action" and promote the idea of "diversity." An important step in developing a personal definition of diversity is thinking about your position on the issue. What is your definition of "diversity"?

Intercultural Communication

Culture is a set of learned behaviors, attitudes, and other things that comprise a way of life. Most likely you share your organization's culture with your co-workers but may not share your personal culture them. Depending on your experience with and exposure to different cultures, your "comfort zone" with different groups can expand or contract.

Miscommunication is a major source of intercultural discomfort and conflict. Communication (verbal, written, and nonverbal) goes beyond what's said, written, or expressed. The process of communicating differs among cultures. Miscommunication can result when an individual's style of communicating differs from that of another person. Your language is part of your culture and binds you to others who speak that language. It can also separate you from those who do not share it. Take care not to let your language create a barrier between you and your co-workers. Instead use your skills to remove barriers and improve communication. If you are bilingual, offer to serve as an interpreter when needed or teach your co-workers some basic words and key phrases for business or for their personal use.

Key Points of Intercultural Communication

- When communications cause conflict, be aware that problems might have more to do with style or process than with content or motives.

- Learn to understand different communication styles. You could benefit through expanding your repertoire.

- Communicating across cultures requires extra effort. Good communication requires commitment and concentration.

- Although culture affects differences in communication patterns, there are many exceptions within each group depending on class, age, education, experience, and personality.

- Remember that communication is a process and that the process varies among cultures. Look at what might be getting in the way of understanding. Constantly ask "What's going on here?" and check your assumptions.

- Avoid jokes, words, or expressions that are hot buttons, such as those that are based on ethnicity, religion, or gender.

- Use language that fosters trust and alliance.

- Respect differences; don't judge people because of the way they speak.

Learning how to communicate among cultures is a necessary ability no matter what type of career you choose. Effective intercultural communication requires you to respect and know how to deal with those differences. Intercultural communication is not easy but there are ways to effectively communicate. These include:

- Respect differences among cultures

- Be flexible

- Do not assume or make judgments

- Be willing to see the other person's point of view

- Give your time and practice intercultural communications.

INTERVIEW QUESTIONS

Federal, state, and local laws regulate the types of questions a prospective employer may ask. Questions asked during the interview and listed on the job application must be related to the job for which you are applying. Questions should address only what the employer needs to know to decide whether or not you can perform the functions of the job. See Figure 10.1. There are several options for answering illegal questions.

- Answer the question, but when choosing to do so realize that you are giving information that is not job related and you could give the "wrong" answer thus, harming your candidacy.

- Refuse to answer the question. You are within your rights, but you risk the chance of being uncooperative or confrontational, therefore, harming your candidacy.

- Examine the intent behind the question and respond with an answer as it might apply to the job. For example, who is going to take care of your children when you have to travel? An appropriate response would be: "I can meet the travel and work schedule that the job requires."

Figure 10.1   Illegal Questions

INQUIRY AREA	ILLEGAL QUESTIONS
National Origin/Citizenship	Are you a U.S. Citizen? Where were you/your parents born? What is your native tongue? Are you authorized to work in the United States? What languages do you read, speak, or write fluently? (Question is okay only if this ability is relevant to the performance of the job.)
Age/Date of Birth	How old are you? What is your birth date? When did you graduate?
Marital/Family Status	What is your marital status? Who do you live with? Do you plan to have a family? When? How many kids do you have? What is the age of your children or dependents? What are your child care arrangements?
Travel	Who will keep your children if you have to travel?
Affiliations	What clubs or social organizations do you belong to? What sorority/fraternity do you belong to?
Personal	How tall are you? How much do you weight? What is your race or color? Is that the real color of your eyes or hair? What is your religion?
Military	Were you honorably discharged from the military?
Disabilities	Do you have any disabilities? What is your medical history? Have you had any recent or past illnesses or operations? How is your family's health? When did you lose your eyesight?
Arrest Record	Have you ever been arrested?

Figure 10.2   Legal Questions

INQUIRY AREA	LEGAL QUESTIONS
Age/personal	Are you over the age of 18?
	Are you able to lift a 50-pound weight and carry it 100 yards, as this is part of the job?
Marital/Family Status Travel	Would you be willing to relocate if necessary?
	Would you be able and willing to travel as needed for the job? (Question is okay if it is asked of all applicants for the job.)
	Would you be able and willing to work overtime as necessary? (Question is okay if it is asked of all applicants for the job.)
Affiliations	What professional or other work related organizations do you belong to?
Military	In what branch of the Armed Forces did you serve?
	What type of training or education did you receive in the military?
Disabilities	Do you have any disabilities that would prohibit you from doing the job?
Arrest Record	Have you ever been convicted of _____?

Adapted from "Handling Illegal Questions" by Rochelle Kaplan (2003), *Planning Job Choices: 2003*, National Association of College and Employers, p. 61.

SUMMARY

Discrimination and harassment issues may be an over-whelming experience for the entry level as well as the experienced employee. When you are mistreated because you are older, pregnant, disabled, your skin color, faith, or sexual orientation it is reassuring to know that you have some legal protections.

Both federal and state laws set out some strict standards on rights and regulations in the workplace. Some of these can be complicated, but worth taking the time to understand. Employers, knowingly or not, may violate these workplace laws, therefore it is necessary for you to be aware of your rights and know where you may go to seek guidance in order to get assistance in resolving these workplace issues.

Your chances of being confronted with discrimination and harassment practices are much less now than was a few years ago. However it's up to you to decide how to handle the situation if one should arise. Employers may or may not lack the knowledge about discrimination and harassment issues but if they do, educate them in a professional manner and follow proper procedures.

REFLECTIONS

1. Read one article or use the Internet to research an issue concerning a liability case about a discrimination or harassment issue. What action did the person take for fail to take? Discuss the outcome of the legal case. What would you have done differently? Use Laboratory 10.1 for your response.

2. Explore a variety of on-line sites related to age, sex, gender, religious, and disability issues on discrimination or harassment. Select two discrimination or harassment issues and based on your research and what would you have done if you were involved in the discrimination or harassment issue as an employer and as an employee. Use Laboratory 10.2 for your response.

WEB SITES

www.aarp.org
American Association of Retired Persons

www.usdoj.gov/crt/ada/adahoml/htm
American With Disabilities Act (ADA)

www.dol.gov
Department of Labor

www.disabilityinfo.gov
Disability Information

www.dol.gov
Family Medical Leave Act (FMLA)

www.asktheinterviewcoach.com
Job Interview Questions.

www.ngltf.org
National Gay and Lesbians

www.nationalpartnership.org
National Partnership for Women and Families

www.pcepd.gov
President's Commission on Employment of People with Disabilities

www.osha.gov
The Occupational Safety and Health Administration (OSHA)

BIBLIOGRAPHY

Clement, A. (1998*). Law In Sport And Physical Activity*. Aurora, Ohio: Sport and Law Press, Inc.

Floyd, P. and Allen, B. (2008). *Professional Preparation Of Pre-Service Teachers*, 2nd ed. Boston, MA: Pearson Education.

Pangrazzi, R.P. and Darst, P.W. (2008). *Dynamic Physical Education For Secondary School Students*, 6th ed. Needham Heights, MA: Pearson Education.

Pangrazi, R. P. (2006*). Dynamic Physical Education For Elementary School Students,* 15th ed. Needham Heights, MA: Pearson Education.

www.careerplanning.about.com
Facts About Pregnancy Discrimination
A Sexual Harassment Primer from the Working Diva at ivillage.com
Pregnancy Rights Knowledge Quiz
Sexual Harassment: What Every Working Woman Needs to Know
FMLA Q & A
Religion in the Workplace
Job Discrimination Cases Reveal Inequity
Age Discrimination
Race Discrimination
Sexual Orientation Discrimination

Religious Discrimination
Religion in the Workplace
Gender Discrimination
National Origin Discrimination
Overtime
When is Disclosure of Your Disability Desirable

www.jobweb.com
ADA, Accommodations, and You
Communicating in the Culturally Diverse Workplace
Key Points of Intercultural Communication
Workplace Culture

www.nolo.com
Nolo.com Legal Encyclopedia: Employees and Contractors
Always on Call? Maybe You Should Be Paid More
Fair Pay and Time Off FAQ
Preventing Sexual Harassment in the Workplace
Sexual Harassment Decisions From the Supreme Court
Sexual Harassment FAQ
Health and Safety FAQ
The Family and Medical Leave Act (FMLA)
Is Carpal Tunnel Syndrome a Disability?

LABORATORY ACTIVITY 10.1

NAME _____ DATE _____

COURSE _____ SECTION _____

Read one article or use the Internet to research a discrimination or harassment issue. What action did the person take or fail to take? Discuss the outcome of the legal case. What would you have done differently?

LABORATORY ACTIVITY 10.2

NAME _____ DATE _____

COURSE _____ SECTION _____

Explore a variety of on-line sites related to age, sex, gender, religious, and disability discrimination or harassment situations. Select two discrimination or harassment issues and based on your research what would you have done if you were involved in the discrimination or harassment issue as an employer and as an employee.